Medicir

Or, The Doctor Scarify'd

Anonymous

Alpha Editions

This edition published in 2022

ISBN : 9789356895201

Design and Setting By
Alpha Editions
www.alphaedis.com
Email - info@alphaedis.com

PREFACE.

IT *being usual for Authors, in Prefaces, to render an Account of the Occasion which gave Birth to their Writings, and to acquaint the Reader with the Design and Scope of their Discourses; I thought it convenient to continue a Custom approved by many illustrious Examples.*

The Motive of publishing this Tract, is not the Intercession of Friends, for none had ever the View of any Part of it; and that it is not Design of Applause that has engaged me in this Undertaking, the Care I have had to conceal my Name will, I suppose, free me from such Suspicion: the chief Inducement proceeds from an Inclination to Mankind, to instruct them to preserve and prolong their Lives, thereby to prevent them from using fraudulent Quack Medicines (which are now become so universally vendible amongst them) or advising with such as are wholly ignorant; and I should think my self sufficiently rewarded for my Pains, if I could arrive to the Point of reforming the Abuses of the present, and restoring the Simplicity of the ancient Practice, by laying open to the World my Observations of the pretended and fallacious Methodus Medendi, *and the Insignificancy of a great Part of their* Materia Medica.

And here I will particularly address my self to all those Persons concern'd with me, who are the People or Patients; and the Physicians with their Followers, the Chirurgeons and Apothecaries: This Discourse is chiefly intended for the first, it being they who are most highly injured by the unwarrantable Practices of those we have therein accused; for although many understanding Persons among the People are sufficiently satisfied of the Abuses we have mentioned; and that it is of absolute Necessity some Reformation should be made: Yet all are not thus perswaded; for we may daily observe, that many who are less discerning, being deceiv'd by an imaginary Good, covet their own Ruin; and unless they be given to understand which is the Evil, and which is the Good, by Persons they have Reason to confide in, they must necessarily run much Hazard.

I have here endeavoured to undeceive them; which I should dispair of, did I only foresee Inconveniencies afar off (the Vulgar being led by Sense, and not by probable Conjectures); but since they do now actually labour under many, and those obvious, Inconveniencies, how short sover their sight be, the Senses of Feeling being no less acute in them than in others, I persuade my self, they will readily assent to those Truths I have largely discovered.

And here must I venture through all the Barricadoes and the Fortifications of popular Resentment; but Satires, like Incision, become necessary when the Humour rankles, and the Wound threatens Mortification; when Advice ceases to work; when Loss, Experience, and Disaster will not convince, then Satire reforms, by making the Error we embrace ridiculous: Shame works to make us forsake a Thing, which Instruction augments, or Persuasion could have no Effect upon.

Many and great Abuses, and of the last Importance to the People, have urged my Duty and demanded my Assistance; and if in my Essay on Health, I do persuade my Reader to the Regimen *I have here laid down, he may assure himself of that* Golden Panacea, *that* Elixir Salutis, *at no other Charge but in* cura seipsum.

It would by many be expected, that I should make an Apology for the great Liberties I have taken in my general Treatment of the whole Faculty; in which I claim the allow'd Exception, that there are some few very Eminent, and worthy of the first Honours and Dignity of Physick, and who by their unwearied Labour of Body and Application of Mind, have run through the Courses of Anatomy, Botany, Chymistry, *and* Galenick Pharmacy, *and no less acquainted with the Virtues, Faults, and Preparations, Compositions and Doses of Vegetables, Animals, Minerals, and all the Shop Medicines.*

And yet nevertheless, the Profession of Physick (though arrived to much greater Improvement than before) it's Dignity and Degrees are so despicably fallen, that the very lowest of People, as well Women as Men, usurp the Title; and how monstrous it is to see that Mob of Empericks, as Barbers, Farriers, and Mountebanks, over-reach and bubble the People both of their Lives and Money.

As I would not arrogate to my self the Performance of another, I must not here forget to acknowledge that I have borrowed from the judicious Author of a late excellent Discourse concerning some few Passages of the State of Physick, and the Regulation of it's Practice. I suppose it will be easily imagined, that I could have spoken the same Things in other Words; but my Respect to the Memory of that worthy Person, disposes me to believe, they will sound better, and be more effectual in his own Language.

The following Appendix receiv'd it's Birth in Answer to some the most formidable of the many Pamphlets that were crowded upon the People at the first Report we had of the miserable State of the Marseillians *by the Plague; which had not been but for the same plausible End, of being serviceable to the Nation, by detecting their Errors, and setting aside the clashing Opinions of those* Literati, *which has rather given Alarm, than a Security to the People.*

To conclude: If in speaking the Truth there is no Blame, but rather Commendation, I then need not Apologise for the Freedom I've used, in exploding the great Varieties and Abuses in both the Theory and Practice of Physick. And although the Attempt should not answer equal to the good Intention I've had for the Publick; yet I shall demand that Justice of the World, and with Horace,

Quod Verum atque decens, curo, & rogo, & omnis in hoc sum.

Medicina Flagellata:
OR, The Doctor Scarify'd.

IT is most certain that all Nations, even the most barbarous, have in all Ages made use of Medicines, to ease their Pains, to regain or preserve Health, the greatest among earthly Felicities; in the Absence whereof, we cannot relish any of those numerous Enjoyments, which the bountiful Creator hath plentifully bestow'd on us; so that the most sublime ancient Philosophers who excluded all other external Good from being necessary, to the well being of Man, placing Happiness only in the things whereof we cannot be depriv'd; yet out of them they excepted Health, knowing there was so near a Connexion between the Soul and Body, that the one could not be disorder'd in its Functions, but the other would be disturb'd in its Operations. Hence it is that no Part of human Knowledge can be of greater Moment than what directs to Remedies, and Means of Relief under those Infirmities to which the whole Race of Man is Heir to; so that even amongst the wisest, that Science or Art whereby those Defects we call Diseases were repair'd, was always accounted Divine; for that God is the first and chief Physician, hath been the constant Faith of all Ages, and that Physicians were accounted the Sons of Gods, was commendably asserted by *Galen*, and therefore it was truly spoken, that Medicines were the Hand of God, there meriting only such Names, as related to their divine Original; thus a certain Antidote was called Ισυθεο, equal to God, another Θεοδοτος, given by God, another divine; several Compositions had the Inscription Ιερα, or Sacred; and 'twas the common Belief among the Heathens, that so great a Knowledge in Physick came by Inspiration: And St. *Austin* is of the same Opinion in his *Civi. Dei*, who saith, *Corporis Medicina (si altius rerum origines repetas) non invenitur unde ad homines manare potuerit, nisi à Deo.* It cannot be conceived whence Physick should come to Man but from God himself.

It is well known how great a Name *Hippocrates* obtain'd, not only in *Greece* (which he deliver'd from the greatest Plague) but in remote Parts; so that the greatest Monarchs of the *East*, and their Vice-Roys, were Suitors to him, to free their Country from that devouring Disease, which threatned to exhaust those populous Regions of their Inhabitants, unless the same Person who freed *Greece* interpos'd, whom they esteem'd divine, and sent from the Gods, because successful in so great Undertakings. Very certain it is, so Noble and Useful a Study were encouraged, yea and practised by Kings, Princes, and Philosophers, by the highest, wisest, and best of Men, whereof some were honour'd by Statues erected to perpetuate their Memoirs, and by many other Instances of the publick Gratitude. So that when I consider what Reverence has been paid to this Profession, and the Professors thereof in all times whereof we have any particular Account, I am amaz'd that in this latter Age wherein it hath received greater Improvements than in Two thousand Years before, and that nevertheless it should be by many neglected, by others slighted, and by some even contemned. After a diligent Enquiry into the Causes of so strange and sudden an Alteration, I could not, in my Opinion, so justly ascribe it to Defects in the Profession, as to those of its Professors; not that I deny that Physick may be capable of greater Improvements, notwithstanding it might to this Day have been maintain'd at least in the same Degree of Honour and Esteem which all Ages have justly had for it, if the Avarice and Imprudence of the Real, the Ignorance and Baseness of the pretended Artists had not interpos'd: Under the former I comprize the Vulgar Physicians; under the latter, their Dependants the Apothecaries, who, I am confident, have caused many of the great Inconveniences under which the Practice of Physick now labours.

That the Sick are in all Cases oppressed with too many Medicines, and made to loath, and complain of the very Cordials; that the Expence is made greater, and more extravagant by the often Confederacy and Artifices visible in the new Modes of prescribing: And the Deaths of the Patient I would not say is frequently the Effect not of the Disease, but of the numerous Doses obtruded in the same Proportions in every Sickness and Age, pushing on declining, and even departing Life; which after its Exit makes Pots and Glasses observed, with the same Passions and Concern, as the bloody Sword is viewed as the Instrument of Death and Mischief. By whom, or by what Means the Purity of Physick has sunk into this Degeneracy, let us farther examine, and trace it from the first Steps of entring into this great Abuse; let us then usher in the young Physician now come from the University, and having spent a great Part of his Money (if not all) in his Education, very wisely for himself considers, which are the most obvious and practis'd Ways of making himself known, and by what Methods he may more easily insinuate himself, and that he may recover the Fortune he has lent the Publick in his Education, which he is resolved they shall now pay him with Interest. He is inform'd, or presently observes, that most, or all the Families are under the Directions of the Apothecary, who gives his Physick 'till he fears the Patient will die, and then appoints a Physician, who before is prepared to acquit him, by bearing the Reproach with the most perfect Resignation. And to support this good Temper, he is bid to cast his Eyes around the Kingdom, and consider how they flourish in the common Fame, who had the good Luck to follow those Instructions at their first Arrival.

Or if he has found out any more effectual Medicines, or more compendious or grateful Methods of Cure, or would imitate the applauded Practice of some few of the most eminent of that Profession, whose Prescriptions were only to assist, not to overload, or suppress Nature; this is too bold a Stroke, a too dangerous Reform in Physick; he must previously consider, that the Number of Apothecaries are increas'd, and that their Dependance lieth more on the Quantities of Medicines in suitable Proportions, and notwithstanding a generous and liberal Education, by which he has learn'd to explode the malevolent and useless Practice, from a great many Prescriptions that are now in vogue; he must not dare to refute them, he must obey that great Principle of Nature, to preserve himself; he must conform to the Manners of the Age, and the general Practice; he must dispence with his not knowing whether the Medicines are made up according to his Prescription; he must wink at the Design, Ignorance, Carelessness, or Unfaithfulness of the Apothecary; whom he must not any ways disgust, tho' he in Revenge, as well in executing his own Interest, may make his Dose up with worm-eaten superannuated Drugs, wherewith most of 'em are well stor'd, which will not work according to the Physician's Promise, and the Patient's Expectation: The Apothecary who here outwits the Doctor, and assumes the Character, is here ready at hand to tell his Patient that this was no ways accommodated to his Temper; nay, perhaps, he presages to him that it will not work sufficiently, (as he may without Conjuring or Astrology) by which he obtains a Reputation of a Person more judicious than the Physician making way for his own Advantage, by telling the Patient that he will prepare a Purge that shall work more effectually than the former: This you need not doubt is the same the Physician before prescrib'd, but assuredly made up of better Drugs, and so the Apothecary executes his Design, which is to exclude the Physician, and prefer himself.

The young Physician, tho' he has learn'd the Abuse, yet he has that Regard to himself, to make use of that old Maxim, *Of the two Evils, to choose the least*; and finding it best suiting his Interest, which otherwise might be endanger'd by the clandestine and underhand Dealings of the other, and now finds it necessary to close in with him, and such a one as will join in a mutual Application and Advancement of each other: Now are their Engines set at work, and the Doctor not to be behind-hand, gives a new Form to his Bills, which he prescribes in Terms so obscure, that he forces all chance Patients to repair to his own Apothecary, pretending a particular Secret, which only they have a Key to unlock; whereas in effect it is no other than the commonest of Medicines disguised under an unusual Name, on design to direct you to that Apothecary, between whom and the Physician there is a private Compact of going Snips out of the most unreasonable Rates of the said Medicines; wherein if you seek a Redress, by shewing the Bill to the Doctor, he shall most religiously aver it to be the cheapest he ever read. The Consequence whereof, as to your Particular, is a double Fraud; and as the Apothecaries in general, their Numbers bearing the Proportion at least ten to one of noted Physicians; to whom allowing his Covenant Apothecary, who constituting one Part of the ten, the remaining nine Parts are compell'd either to sit still, or to quack for a Livelihood, or at least eight of them, for we'll suppose one Part of the nine a Possibility of acquiring competent Estates, in a Way more honest than that of the Covenanters, by their wholsome Trade of fitting out Chirurgeons Chests for Sea, and supplying Country Apothecaries with Compositions: Lastly, all accomplish'd Physicians are likewise expos'd to manifest Injuries from the Covenant Apothecaries, who being sent for by Patients, after a short Essay of a Cordial, will overpower them by Perswasions to call in a Doctor, who shall be no other than his Covenant Physician; by which Means the former Physician, who by his extraordinary Care and Skill had oblig'd the Family before, shall be passed by, and lose the Practice of that Patient: And should it happen, the Sense of Gratitude of the forementioned Patient, should engage him to continue the Use of his former Physician, yet this Covenant Apothecary shall privately cavil at every Bill, and impute the Appearance of every small Pain, or Symptom (which necessarily in the Course of a Disease will happen) to his ill Address in the Art of Physick, and shall not give over before he has introduc'd his Covenanter, whose Authority in the Fraud of Physick he supposes to be most necessary.

But least you should think me overbalanc'd with a Prejudice to those that so much abuse that noble Profession, I'll conduct you into their usual Road and Method of examining their Patients, and making Enquiry into their Diseases, wherewith being acquainted, you may, without any farther Conviction, pronounce a Verdict.

This Knack doth chiefly consist in three Notions; *viz. First,* That a Patient's Grievance is either a discernible evident Disease, which his own Confession makes known to you, what it is; or, *Secondly*, an inward Pain; or, *Thirdly*, one of those two Endemic Diseases, a Scurvy, or Consumption; or, a *Fourth*, the Pox. This is their Theory, which is so deeply ingrafted on their *Dura Mater*, and may be acquired with less Industry than fourteen Years Study at one of our Universities; for so much Time is requir'd to make a Man grow up a Doctor, the Formality whereof in most Places consists in this Elogy; *Accipiamus pecuniam, & dimittamus asinùm.*

If a sick Man makes his Address to a vulgar Physician, he demands his Complaint; t'other replies, he is troubled either with a Vomiting, Looseness, want of Stomach, Cough, bad Digesture, difficulty of Breathing, a Phtisick, Faintness, Jaundice, Green-Sickness, Dropsy, Gout, Convulsion-Fits, Palsy, Diziness, or Swimming in the Brain, Spitting of Blood, an Ague, a continual great Heat or Fever, *&c.* These are all evident Diseases the Party himself expresses he is troubled with; but his Sickness not being an evident Disease, which he himself can explain, the Vulgar Doctor concludes, it must be either an inward Pain, or an Endemick Disease: The Patient then making complaint of an inward Pain, to his old way of guessing t'other goes, enquiring first in what Part? If he answers, he feels a Pain in the right Side, or under the short Ribs, he tells him it is an Obstruction, or Stoppage in the Liver; if in the left Side, in the opposite Part, then 'tis a Stoppage of the Spleen; if in the Belly, he it may be calls it a Cholick, or Wind in the Guts; if in the Back, or Loins, he perswades him it's Gravel, Stone, or some other Obstruction in the Kidneys; if a Stitch in the Breast, he terms it Wind, or other times a Pleurisy: Lastly, if the Party be reduc'd to a very lean Carcass, by reason of a long tedious Cough, Spitting of Blood, or want of Stomach, or Feebleness, or almost any other Disease, or Pain, then besure he tells him he's in a Consumption, or at least falling into one: But being troubled with several Diseases and Pains at once, as running Pains, Faintness, want of Stomach, change of Complexion, so as to look a little yellowish, duskish, or greenish; then t'other whispers him, he is troubled with the Scurvy. If diseased with Ulcers or running Sores, red, yellow, blue, or dark Spots, Pimples, or Blotches in the Face, Arms, Legs, or any other Part of the Body, that's determin'd to be the Scurvy likewise, supposing the Party to be a sober discreet Person: But if appearing inclined to Wantonness by reason of his Youth, or sly Countenance, then the fore-mention'd Disease is to be call'd the Pox. In most Diseases of Women, they accuse the Mother. In Children, their Guess seems far more fallible; for a Child within the six Months being taken ill, restless, and froward, if there appear no evident Disease, he ever affirms it's troubled with Gripes; upon which he prognosticates, that if not speedily remedied, the Child will fall into Convulsion-Fits; but this not happening according to his Prediction, to prevent the Forfeiture of his Skill and Repute, endeavours to possess the Mother, and rest of the Gossips, it had inward Fits. The Child being past six Months, and falling indispos'd, then instead of Gripes, it is discompos'd by breeding of Teeth; but having bred all his Teeth, and being surpriz'd with any kind of Illness, the Doctor then avouches it is troubled with Worms: In short, take away these three Words, Obstruction, Consumption, and Scurvy, and there will remain three dumb Doctors, the Hackney Physician, the Prescribing Surgeon, and the Practicing Apothecary.

Hitherto we have only discovered to you the Ordinary Physicians conjecturing Compass, whereby he steers his Course, to arrive to the Knowledge of his Patients Diseases: There yet remains we should unlock the other Ventricle of his Brain, to behold the Subtilty of his Fancy in groaping at the Causes of Diseases, which, tho' the Poet declares (*Felix qui potuit rerum cognoscere causas*) to be cloathed with the darkest Clouds, yet by the Virtue of this following Principle, aims at this Mark immediately, *viz.* That most Diseases are caus'd by Choler, Phlegm, Melancholy, or abundance of Blood: Of these, two are suppos'd to be hot, namely, Choler, and abundance of Blood, and the other two cold, to wit, Phlegm, and Melancholy, and consequently Causes of hot and cold Diseases: These four Universals being reduced to two general Categories; under the Notion of hot and cold, any one having but the Sense of distinguishing Winter from Summer, may, in the Time of an *Hixius Doxius*, instantly appoint a Cause for almost every Disease: So that a Patient discovering his Trouble, it may be a want of Stomach, bad Digesture, Fainting, Cough, Difficulty of breathing, Giddiness, Palsy, *&c.* his Vulgar Physician has no more to do, but take him by the Fist, to feel whether he be hot or cold; if he finds him cold, then summons in his old Causes, Phlegm, and Melancholy; which ready, and quick pronouncing of the Cause upon a meer Touch, doth almost stupify your Patient, thro' Admiration of *Æsculapian* Oracle, hitting him in the right Vein to a hair's breadth: For, quoth he, indeed, Mr. Doctor, I think you understand my Distemper exceedingly well, and have infallibly found out the Cause; for every Morning as soon as I awake, I spit such a deal of Phlegm, and moreover, I must confess my self extreamly given to Melancholy. This jumping in Opinions between them, makes Mr. Doctor swell with Expectation of a large Fee, which the Patient most freely forces on him, and so the Fool and his Monies are soon parted. Now it's two to one but both are disappointed, the one in his unexperienced Judgment, t'other in his fond Belief; for, state the Case, the Disease takes its Growth from Choler, or abundance of Blood, or any other internal Cause; there is scarce one in a hundred that are indispos'd, who is not subject to hauk and spit in the Morning, and being reduc'd to Weakness, by reason of his Trouble, must necessarily be heavy in the Passions of the Mind, and incident to melancholy Thoughts, through the Memory of his Mortality, occasion'd by this Infirmity: So that, seldom Mirth and Cheerfulness are housed in indispos'd Bodies, because they are deficient of that abundance of Light, and clear Spirits, required to produce them. No Wonder the Vulgar is so opinionated in the Affair of their Temperament, when belabour'd with a Disease; since in their healthful State, it's impossible for a Physician to engage their Opinion otherwise, than to believe themselves phlegmatick and melancholy.

To return to the Point of declaring how the Vulgar strives even with Violence to be cheated, not in their Purses only, but in their Fancies and Opinion; and in this Particular, our Women are so violent eager, that if the Vulgar Physician can but make a true Sound upon the Treble of their Fancy, will produce such a Harmony as shall sound his Praise through City and Country; and without those Female-Instruments, or She-Trumpets, it's almost impossible for a Vulgarist to arrive to a famous Report, who having once by his Tongue-Harmony inchanted the Woman, doth by the same Cheat subject the Opinion of Man to his Advantage, Women generally usurping, and impropriating the Affair of their Husbands Health to their own Management; for if a Man chance to be surpriz'd with Sickness, he presently asks his Wife what Doctor he shall send to, who instantly gives her Direction to him that had her by the Nose last. In this Piece of Subtilty, the Doctor shews him self no less cunning than the Serpent in *Genesis*, who, to cheat *Adam*, thought it expedient first to deceive *Eve.*

Now without any further Preamble, I must tell you the Humour many a sick Woman delights to be coaks'd in by the Ordinary Physician, *viz.* She loves to be told she is very melancholy, tho' of never so merry a Composure, and in that Part of the Litany, Mr. Doctor is a perfect Reader; for a Woman making Complaint she is troubled with Drowsiness, want of Stomach, Cough, or any other Distemper; he answers her, she is in an ill State, and troubled with great and dangerous Diseases, and all engender'd by Melancholy; and then tells her over again, she is very melancholy, and, saith he, probably occasion'd by coarse Treats at Home, or some Unkindness of Friends, which makes the poor Heart put Fingers in her Eye, and force a deep Sigh or two; and all this possibly for being deny'd the extravagant Charge of a Tea-Equipage, or a new Gown on a *May*-Day; which being refresh'd in her Memory, doth certainly assure her, the Impression of that Melancholy to be the Original of her Trouble, tho' some Months or Years past, especially since her Physician discovers to her so much: And for so doing, admires him no less, intending withal to give him an ample Testimony to the World of the Doctor's great Skill: But this is not all, he pursues his Business, looks into her Eyes, where 'spying a small Wrinkle or two in the inward or lesser Angle, he tells her, she has had a Child or two, namely, a Boy, or a Girl, according to the Place of the aforesaid Wrinkle in the right or left inward Angle; thence perswades her, that at her last lying in, her Midwife did not perform her Office skilfully, or did not lay her well, whereby she receiv'd a great deal of Prejudice, as Cold, Wrenching, displacing of the *Matrix*, &c. Which Instance squaring with the premeditated Sense and Opinion of his She-Patient, (most Women, though never so well accommodated in their Labour, being prone to call the Behaviour of their Midwife in Question) he hath now produced a far greater Confidence than before: And last of all, to compleat his Work now at the going off of his gull'd Patient, of rendring her Thoughts, Opinion, and Confidence, Vassals to his Service, Fame, and Advantage, makes one Overture more, of a great Cause of some of her Symptoms, declaring to her, she is much subject to Fits of the Mother, occasioning a Choaking in her Throat, and herein they also jump in their Sentiments; scarce one Woman in an hundred but one time or other is assaulted by those Uterin Steams, especially upon a Tempest of any of the Passions of Fright, Fret, Anger, Love, *&c.*

If I have reproached the Vulgar Physician for executing his Employ with so little Ingenuity, far greater Reason may move me to condemn the Water-gazer, who by the Steams of the Urine, pretends to gratify his Patient's nice Curiosity, of being resolv'd what was, what is, and what Disease is to come;

and what is more, some by their great Cunning aiming to discover as much by the Urinal, as the Astrologer by the Globe. The Fame unto which the *English* Doctor, who some Years ago residing at *Leyden*, promoted himself by his wonderful Sagacity in Urins, is not unworthy of your Note, hundreds, or rather thousands repairing to this stupendious Oracle, to have the State of their Bodies describ'd by Urine. But when I relate to you the first Means that gave Birth to our Countryman's Repute, I shall soon remove your Passion of admiring him. Upon his Arrival at the Place aforemention'd, he had in his Company a bold Fellow, that haunted the most noted Taverns and Tap-houses, who by way of Discourse divulg'd the good Fortune that was happened to the Town, by the Arrival of an *English* Doctor, whose great Learning, and particular Skill in Urins, would soon render him famous to all the Inhabitants. This being pronounced with a Confidence suitable to the Subject, occasion'd three sick Scholars (two Hecticks, one Hydropical) then present, to make Trial of the Truth of his Words; the next Morning, agreeing to mix all their Urins in one Urinal, and commit the Carriage of it to him that was dropsical. In the Interim, the Doctor advertis'd of it by his Companion, which made him so skilful, that when the Hydropical Scholar presented him with the Urinal, to know the State of his diseased Body, he soon gravely reply'd, that he observed three Urins in this one Urinal, whereof the two lowermost Parts of the Urin, appear'd to him to be consumptive, and the third that floated at top dropsical, and with all, that their Conditions were desperate, and at the Expiration of six Months they should be all lodg'd in their Graves. This admirable Dexterity of discerning Diseases by the Urinal, was soon proclaim'd by the Scholars themselves, who all having finish'd the Course of their Lives, within the Time prefix'd, proved an undoubted Argument of his unparallel'd Parts in the Art of Physick, which immediately procur'd him an incredible Concourse of People for many Years together.

Another Instance of a Woman whose Husband had a Bruise by a Fall down Stairs, carry'd his Urin to the Urin casting Doctor in *Moor-fields*, who pretended likewise to be a Conjurer; he (after shaking) seeing little Specks of Blood float in it, had so much Understanding to tell her, that the Party had receiv'd some internal Hurt; the Woman agreed to this as Truth, but demanding by what Means he came by it: Upon this he erected a Scheme, and in the mean time asked her so many Questions, that by the Drift of her Discourse, he gather'd that he had tumbled down Stairs: The Woman not minding well what she had said, (in the Consternation she was in at the hard Words he had utter'd) suppossing he was conjuring up the Devil, to be resolv'd in the Matter, told her own Words in a different Title; the Woman acknowledged it true, with some Admiration, but desir'd to know how many Pair of Stairs he might fall down? She had told him before where she liv'd (and he considering the Place chiefly consisted of low Buildings) answer'd, two Pair. Nay, now said she, you are out in your Art, he fell three Story I'll promise. This put our Doctor to his Trumps, when having mused a while for an Excuse, he shook the Urinal again, and asked her if there was all the Water her Husband had made? No, reply'd she, I spilt a little in pouring it in. O ho, did you so? said he: Why that, Woman, was the Business that made me mistake, for there went away the other Pair of Stairs in the Urin you spilt.

I shall but trouble you with another Instance, which explodes this Cheat, of what happened in the early Practice of the fam'd Dr. *Radcliff* when at *Oxford*; of a Country Woman that brought to him her Husband's Urin in a Glass-Bottle, very carefully cork'd up; and after a low Courtesy, presented the Bottle, desiring the Doctor to send a Remedy for her Husband, who then lay very ill: The Doctor observing the Simplicity of this Woman, put no other Question, but of what Profession or Trade her Husband was of? Who reply'd, a Shoemaker: At which he pours forth the Urin in a Basin then by him, and after he had supply'd it with a like Quantity of his own, he gives it her, and says, Good Woman, carry this to your Husband, and bid him fit me with a Pair of Boots: but she replying, Her Husband must first take Measure; to which he return'd, The Shoemaker might as well judge by the Urinal the fitting of his Leg, as he in that of his Distemper. That the Effects of Confederacy in promoting a Physician to a popular Vogue, are as powerful as sinister and disingenuous, may not only be deduced from the aforesaid Naratives, but from the common Design of vulgar Empericks, who to raise their Fame as high as a Pyramid, send forth several prating Fellows into all publick Places, Taverns, Coffee-houses, and Ale-houses, to publish their vast Abilities, expecting with that Bait to hook in as many Patients as will swallow it. Others are no less skill'd in counterfeiting their great Practice, by causing their Apothecaries, or others, to call them out of the Church at an Afternoon Sermon, to hasten Post to a suborn'd Patient, to the Intent the World be advertis'd of the weighty Business this Doctor is concern'd in. Others by their Equipage, eminent Houses, and occasioning one and the same Patient, to repair needlesly to them twenty or thirty times, manifest a Decoy even taken Notice of by the Vulgar. These few disingenuous Ways, do here purposely bring on Board, omitting many others, to convince the Publick, that the only Means for a Physician to advance himself honourably to Practice, is by discovering his real Abilities in curing Diseases, by quick, certain, and pleasant Medicines; and therefore nothing should render his Parts more suspicious than by attempting their Discovery by such fallacious and ignoble Devices; for certainly the Conclusion is most sophistical, that because this Doctor is drawn in his Coach, t'other rides on Horseback, or another hath his Lacquey at his Heels, therefore he must be excellently qualify'd in his Profession, but *Vulgus vult decipi.*

If I now describe, by way of Advice to those that are entering upon the Study of this divine Art, the Method of attaining to a Point of Excellency in it, and that may serve our Vulgar for a better Rule to distinguish their Qualifications by the Course they have passed through; for it is most necessarily requisite, our young Student should be perfectly instructed in the *Latin* and *Greek* Tongues, being the Universal Keys to unlock all those Arts and Sciences, and no less a Grace to the future Physicians. In this Particular, many of our Embryonated Physicians, that have of late Years transported themselves to *Leyden*, and *Utrecht*, to purchase a Degree, have been found very defective; insomuch, that I have heard the Professors condemn several of them for their shameful Imperfection in that which is so great an Ornament, and of so absolute an Use in the Study of Physick: Neither can less be suspected of some of the more aged Vulgar Physicians, making Choice to manage their Consultations in the Vulgar Tongue. *Secondly*, Being thus qualify'd for a Student, he ought to apply himself close to the Study of Phylosophy, for which, *Oxford* and *Cambridge* may justly challenge a Pre-eminence above other Universities: Here it is our Student learns to speak like a Scholar, and is inform'd in the Principles of Nature, and the Constitutions of Natural Bodies; and so receiving a rough Draught in his Mind, is to be accomplish'd by that excellent Science of Human Bodies. But because, according to the first Aphorism of the first Master *Hippocrates*, Art is long, and Life short, he ought to engage his Diligence to absolve his Philosophical Course in two Years at longest, and in the interim, for his Recreation and Divertisement, enter himself Scholar to the Gardiner of the Physick-Garden, to be acquainted with the Fœtures of Plants, but particularly with those that are familiarly prescrib'd by Practitioners, to prevent being outwitted by Herb-women in the Markets, and to enable him to give a better Answer, than is said once of a Physician, who having prescrib'd *Maiden-hair* in his Bill, the Apothecary asked which Sort he meant; t'other reply'd, some of the Locks of a Virgin. *Thirdly*, Supposing our Student having made sufficient Progress in Philosophy, may now pass to *Leyden*, and may enter himself into a *Collegium Anatomicum*, Anatomy being the Basis and Foundation whereon the weighty Structure of Physick is to be raised; and unless he acquires more than ordinary Knowledge and Dexterity in this, will certainly be deceiv'd in the Expectation of ever arriving to the Honour of an accomplish'd Physician: A Proficiency in that Part fits him for a *Collegium Medicum Institutionum*, and afterward for a *Collegium Practicum*, and then 'tis requisite he should embrace the Opportunity of visiting the Sick in the Hospital twice a Week with the Physick-Professor, where he shall examine those Patients with all the Exactness imaginable, and point at every Disease, its Symptoms, as it were, with his Fingers, and afterward propose several Cases upon those Distempers, demanding from every young Student his Opinion, and his Grounds, and his Reasons for it; withal requiring of him what Course of Physick is best to be prescrib'd: This is the only Way for a young Physician to attain a Habit of knowing Diseases when he seeth them; and a confident

Method of curing those that may repair to him, without running the Hazard of being censured by Apothecaries, or derided by them for his Bills, as too many are, that at *Oxford* or *Cambridge* have only imbib'd a Part of *Senuert*'s Institutions, and overlook'd *Riverius*'s Practice, and thence attaining an imperfect and unhappy Skill, by enlarging the Church-yards in the City or Country; but what is more, he shall escape the Danger a young Student I formerly knew at *Oxford* precipitated himself into, by imagining every Disease he read was his own. I must likewise advise our Student to take his Lodgings there at an able Apothecary's House, to contract the Knowledge of Drugs, and of preparing, dispensing, and mixing them in Compositions, and then by Means of his own Qualifications, may boldly pretend to inform, correct, and improve those Apothecaries which the Chance of his Practice shall conduct him to; for it would be judged ridiculous, should a Physician undertake to reprehend, and afterwards bend his Force to suppress and decry Apothecaries privately or publickly, without having first acquired a particular Experience in their Art. Hence it is again the Vulgar Physician is wrapped up in a Cloud, and the Apothecaries dance round about him; he prescribes Medicines he never saw; they prepare them according to their own Will and Pleasure.

Neither is it over these alone the Physician claims a Superintendance, but over Chirurgeons likewise; and therefore in this his Course of Study, would contribute to his future Qualifications, in sojourning a Year with some experienc'd manual Operator, without a Hindrance to his other Affair, and there by an ocular Inspection, and handling of his Instruments, demanding their Names, Uses, and Manner of using, withal by Insinuations to visit the Chirurgical Patients, and see him dress them, would render his Study in Chirurgery, so plain and easy, which otherwise might be thought difficult, that it should enable him to give Laws to Chirurgeons also, especially to those that execute their Office with that Rashness, Indiscretion and Dishonesty as I have sometime discover'd amongst them.

These two Years giving occasion to our Student to acquire a System, or a brief Comprehension of the Theory of Physick, and of the Practice likewise: Nothing now remains than to amplify his commenc'd Knowledge and Experience by his farther Travels; to which End, takes his Journey to *Paris*, to be acquainted with the most famous Physicians, and to be inform'd of their Way of Practice, by surveying their Prescripts at the most frequented Apothecaries, to visit for a Year every Day the Hospitals of *l'Hostel Dieù*, and *la Charitè*; in which latter, it is customary, for any three or four young Physicians to examine and overlook the new enter'd Patients, to name the Distempers among themselves, and propose their Cures, for to compare their Opinions afterwards with the Physicians that are appointed for the Hospital, and where he may see most difficult Operations perform'd in

Chirurgery, as Trypaning, Amputating, Cutting for the Stone, Tapping of the Belly and Breast with the greatest Dexterity. Here he may also observe Wounds and Ulcers cured by Virtue of those famed Waters, *viz.* the White Water, and the Yellow Water; the former being *Aqua Calcis*, the latter the same, with an Addition of *Sublimate.*

The Art of preparing Medicines chymically, having merited a great Esteem for its stupendious and admirable Effects in the most despair'd Diseases, shews a Necessity of being instructed in it, in which he can not fail of prying into, in the Course of his Travels.

Having attained his Scope in this Place, his Curiosity ought to direct him to *Montpellier*, where he will meet with a Concourse of the greatest Proficients in Physick in *Europe*, converse with the Professors and Physicians of that Place, and out of 'em all, extract choice Observations, Secrets, and most subtle Opinions upon several Diseases, which Design can scarce be compassed in less than another Year. Now we must suppose our Student to merit the Title of an experienc'd Physician, and raised far above the Vulgar ones, that never felt the Cold beyond the Chimneys of their own Homes: He is now render'd capable of understanding the greatest Mysteries, and most acute Opinions in Physick, which he is chiefly to expect from those reputed Professors of the *Albò* at *Padua*, where he is likewise to continue his Diligence in visiting the famed Hospital of *San Lorenzo*, and observe the *Italian* Method of curing Diseases by alterative Broths, without purging or bleeding, that Climate seldom suffering Plethories in those dry Bodies: He cannot but be wonderfully pleased with the Variety and excellent Order of the Plants of their Physick Garden, by them call'd *Horto di Sempleci.* Neither will he receive less Satisfaction from the curious and most dextrous Dissections perform'd by the artificial Hand of the Anatomy Professor. Having here made his Abode for six Months, may justly aspire to a Degree of a Doctor in Physick, which the Fame of the Place should persuade him to take here, being the Imperial University for Physick of all others in the World, and where Physicians do pass a very exact Scrutiny, and severe Test. Hence may he transport himself to *Bologn*, and in three Months time add to his Improvements what is possible by the Advantage of the Hospital, and the Professors. Last of all, in the Imitation of the diligent Bee sucking Honey out of all sweet Flowers, our Doctor must not neglect to extract something that his Knowledge did not partake of before, out of the eminentest Practitioners at *Rome*, examine the chief Apothecaries Files, and still frequent those three renown'd Hospitals of *San Spirito* in the *Vatican*, *San Giovanni Laterano* on the Mount *Celio*, and that of *San Giacomo di Augusta* in the Valley *Martia*, besides many others of less Note.

Here may he see the Rarities and Antiquities of this once renowned Empress of the World, from whence he may visit the renowned City of *Naples*, and take a Survey of the Antiquities of the Nature of *Pazzoli*.

Having thus in all Particulars satisfied his Curiosity, may consult about the most advantageous Ways homeward, which is to embark for *Leghorn*, or *Genoa*, where he cannot fail of *English* Shipping.

Or else may take a Tour by Land to *Milan*, where he will see the finest Hospital, and the strongest Citadel in *Europe*. Hence passes the *Alpes*, and that stupendous Mount St. *Godart*, through *Altorph*, and *Lucern*, and thence to *Bazil*, the chief of the Protestant *Cantons*, so by Boat down the River *Rhine* to *Strasburgh*, and *Heydelbergh*, *Manheim*, and so down the *Rhine* to *Coblentz*, *Audernach* and *Collen*, then by Land to *Brussels*, *Ghant*, *Ostend*, *Newport*, and *Dunkirk*, *Gravelin*, and *Calais*: And thence to the Place of his Inclinations for his future Settlement, where, by his vast Experience and Knowledge, being render'd conspicuous in the secure and certain Method of his Cures, will soon give Occasion to the People to discern the Difference between him and the ordinary vulgar Physicians, who by their sordid Deports, and dangerous Practice, make it their Business to ease the blind People of the Weight in their Pockets, and plague them in worse Diseases.

How very few go through this Course of Improvement, we too readily discover, and may be reproved by the first beginning of the Practice among the Ancients, where we find the Method then in use, to train up Youth to the Profession, was to place them Apprentices with able Physicians, who adjudged it necessary to take their Beginning from Surgery, the Subject whereof being external Diseases, as Wounds, Swellings, Members out of joint, and others that were visible, proved more facile and easy to their inmate Capacities, and wherein they might suddenly become serviceable to their Masters, in easing them of the Trouble of dressing and cleansing stinking Ulcers, and applying Ointments and Plaisters, a nauseous Employ, which they ever endeavour'd to abandon to their Scholars with what Expedition possible: This as it was the easiest, so it was the first, and ancientest Part of Physick, and from which those that exercised it were anciently not called Surgeons, but Physicians, tho' they attempted no other Diseases but what were external; according to which Sense *Æsculapius* the first Physician, or Inventor of Physick, and his Sons *Podalyrius* and *Machaon*, are by History asserted to have undertaken only those that wanted external Help; internal Diseases being in those Days unknown, and by Temperance in their Diet, wholly debarr'd; and if accidentally an internal Distemper did surprize them, they apply'd a general Remedy (having no other) of poisoning or killing themselves with a Dagger or Sword, thereby chusing rather to die once, and finish their Misery, than to survive the Objects of Peoples Pity, or to endure the Shocks of Death by every Pain or Languor, especially since the sage

Judgment of that Age did esteem it a signal Virtue to despise and scorn the vain World, by hurrying out of it in a Fury, a Maxim most of the Philosophers were very eminent in observing; and was likewise extended to Children that brought any Diseases external or internal with them into the World, their Cure being perform'd immediately by strangling, or drowning them; neither was this Art of external Physick of short Continuance; *Pliny* writing that Six hundred Years after the building of *Rome*, the *Romans* entertain'd Chyrurgical Physicians from *Peloponesus*: Idleness and Gluttony at last exchang'd their Ease into a Disease, which soon put them into a Necessity of experimenting such Remedies as might re-establish them into that healthful Condition, which Exercise in War, and Temperance in Diet had for so many Ages preserved their Ancestors in.

Upon a competent Improvement of their Scholars in this external Practice of Physick, and their deserving Deportment, they thought them worthy of giving them Entrance into their Closets, to be instructed in such Matters as the most retir'd Places of their Cabinets contained; which were their Remedies and Medicines, and the Manner of preparing them: And then bending his Endeavours to arrive to the Art of discerning the Disease by its Signs, and making Observations upon the Prognosticks, all critical and preternatural Changes: The Dose, Constitution, and all other Circumstances of giving the Medicines which he did gradually accomplish, by his sedulous Attendance on his Master, and his practical Discourses and Lectures from him on every Patient he visited: Lastly, upon his Attainment to a Degree of Perfection in the Art, discovered by his Master by his private Examination, all the Physicians and Commonalty of the Place were summoned to be present at the taking of his Oath in the publick Physick-School, which served in lieu of making Free to Practise, or taking his Degree; the Form of which, as remarkable as it is ancient, the Oath was as followeth.

"I Swear by [1]*Apollo* the Physician, and [2]*Æsculapius*, and by [3]*Hygea*, and [3]*Panacea*, and I do call to witness all the Gods, and likewise all the Goddesses, that according to my Power and Judgment I will entirely keep this Oath and this Covenant; That I will esteem this Master that taught me this Art, give him his Diet, and with a thankful Spirit, impart to him whatever he wants; and those that are born of him I will esteem them as my Male Brethren, and teach them this Art, if they will learn it, without Hire or Agreement; I will make Partakers of the Teaching, Hearing, and of all the whole Discipline, my own and my Master's Sons, and the rest of the Disciples, if they were bound before by Writing, and were obliged by the Physicians Oath, no other besides; I will, according to my Capacity and Judgment, prescribe a Manner of Diet suitable to the Sick, free from all Hurt or Injury; neither will I, through any bodies Intercession, offer Poison to any, neither will I give Counsel to any such Thing; neither will I give a Woman a

Pessary to destroy her Conception: Moreover, I will exercise my Art, and lead the rest of my Life chastly and holily; neither will I cut those that are troubled with the Stone, but give them over to Artists that profess this Art; and whatever Houses I shall come into, I will enter for the Benefit of the Sick; and I will abstain from doing any voluntary Injury, from all Corruption, and chiefly from that which is venereal, whether I should happen to have in Cure the Bodies either of Women or of Men, or of free-born Men or Servants; and whatever I shall chance to see or hear in curing, or to know in the common Life of Men; if it be better not to utter it, I will conceal, and keep by me as Secrets: That as I entirely keep and do not confound this Oath, it may happen to me to enjoy my Life and my Art happily, and celebrate my Glory among all Men to all Perpetuity; but if transgressing and forswearing, that the contrary may happen."

Between those Bounds of Secresy, Veneration, Honesty and Gratitude, the Art was for many hundred Years maintained; for in the Time of *Galen*, and many Ages after him, Medicines for their greater Secresie were used to be prepared and composed by Physicians, as you may read, *Libr. de Virt. Centaur.* where is observable, their Men were wont to carry their Physick ready prepar'd in Boxes after them, which they themselves, according to the Exigency, did dispense. This Custom was continued until Wars ceasing, People began to be as intent upon the Propagation of Mankind, as the Cruelty of the former martial Ages had been upon its Destruction; where the World growing numerous, and through Idelness and want of those Diversions of their military Employ, addicting themselves to Gluttony, Drunkenness, and Whoredom, did contract so great a Number of all inward Diseases, that their Multiplicity imposed a Necessity upon Physicians (being unable to attend them all as formerly) to dismember their Act into three Parts, whereof two were servile, Chirurgery and Pharmacy; and the other imperial and applicative or methodical.

The servile Part being now committed to such as are now called Surgeons and Apothecaries, the former were employed in applying external Medicines to external Diseases; the latter in preparing all ordinary internal and external Medicines, according to the Prescription and Directions of the Physicians, whose Servants were ordered to fetch the prescrib'd Medicines at the Apothecaries, and thence to convey them to their Patients; by which Means the Apothecary was kept in Ignorance: As to the Application and Use of the said Medicines, not being suffered to be acquainted with the Patients or their Diseases, to prevent their Insinuation into their Acquaintance, which otherwise might endanger the diverting the said Patients to other Physicians, or at least their presuming themselves to venture at their Distempers. Neither were the Physicians Servants in the least Probability of undermining or imitating their Masters in the Practice, not knowing their Medicines or

Prescriptions. Besides all this, those Remedies from which the chief Efficacy and Operation against the Disease was expected, still remain'd secret with the Physicians, who thought it no Trouble to prepare them with their own Hands. Thus you may remark the Physician's necessary Jealousy of their Underlings, and their small Pains prov'd the sole Means of impropriating their Art to themselves: And yet by the Advantage of their Chirurgeons and Apothecaries, were capacitated to visit and cure ten times greater Numbers of Sick than before; which in a short Time improved their Fame and Estate to a vast Treasure, whence it was well rhimed,

——*dat Galenus Opes, dat Justinianus Honores.*

But at length, their Honour and vast Riches in the Eye of Apothecaries and Surgeons, proved Seeds sown in their Minds, that budded into Ambition of becoming Masters, and into Covetousness of Equality, and shareing with them in their Wealth; both which they thought themselves capable of aspiring to by an Emperical Skill the Neglect and Sloath of their Masters had given them occasion to attain, since they did not begin to scruple to make them Porters of their Medicines to their Patients, to intrust them with the Preparation of their greatest Secrets. This Trust they soon betray'd, for having insinuated into a familiar Acquaintance with their Masters Patients, it was a Task not difficult to perswade them, that those that had made and dispensed the Medicines, were as able to apply them to the like Distempers, as they that had prescrib'd them, who had either forgot, or were wholly ignorant how to prepare them; so that now they were as good as arrived to a Copartnership with their Masters in Reputation and Title, the best being call'd Doctors alike, and there being no other Difference between them, than that the Master Doctor comes at the Heells of his Man Doctor, to take in Hand the Work which he or his Brother Doctor (the Chirurgeon) had either spoiled, or could not farther go on with; a very fine Case the Art of Physick and its Professors are reduc'd to, and that not only of late Days, but of almost Seven hundred Years, for before that time Apothecaries had scarce a Being, only there were those they call'd *Seplasiarij* from their selling of Ointments on the Market of *Capua*, call'd *Seplasia*, *Armatarij*, and *Speciarij*, or such as sold Drugs and Spices; tho' I confess Apothecaries may offer a just Objection in pretending to a far greater Antiquity, since the Original and Necessity of their Employ was deriv'd from the *Egyptian* Bird *Isis*, spouting Water into its Breech for a Glyster: But 'tis no Matter, the Doctor must truckle to this powerful Engineer, he must conform to the Manner of the Age; and were I to enumerate the many Abuses that are practised by this lower Profession, I mean the Generality of them, you would be more careful in making Choice of your Apothecary, or making a better Choice in having least to do with them; and how dangerous is their Ignorance in the *Latin* Tongue, which is of very ill Consequence, as their Prescriptions sent 'em by the Physicians are writ in *Latin*, and which not being rightly understood, hath often occasioned not only innocent but fatal Mistakes. *Homine semi docto quid iniquius?* and that a great Part of the Apothecaries are very illiterate! is so evident, that they themselves dare not deny it; among many Instances of this Kind, that most unfortunate one recorded by an eminent Physician is notorious, who instead of a Dose of *Mercurius sublimatus dulcis*, exhibited so much common Sublimate, a mortal Poison, which was scarce ever given inwardly, instead of an innocent Medicine approved by all Physicians. Yet those worthy Sons of Bombast must disgust your Palate with the Relation of the nauseous and choaking Terms, their Ends of *Latin* and stifling Phrases, driving to confound and amaze the simple Vulgar. An Instance of this Kind may afford you some little Diversion: A practical Apothecary coming to see his Customer, a Cobler, that lay indisposed of the Cholick, observed him to crack a Fart (for so it is express'd in the Original) upon which, said the Apothecary, Sir, that's nothing but the Tonitruation of Flatuosities in your Intestines; this was no sooner out of his Mouth, but the Cobler crack'd another, and reply'd to his Doctor, Sir, that is nothing but your Hobgoblin Notes thundring Wind out of my Guts; which literal Return of his Terms of Art in plain *English*, though by chance, obliged the Apothecary to this Expression; I beg your Pardon, Sir, I suppose you have study'd the Art of Physick as well as my self, and want not my Help: So away went Doctor Pestle, imagining the Cobler to be as great a Master in the Faculty as himself.

Another Complaint against the Apothecaries is, That they are not well acquainted with the *Materia Medica*; the Knowledge of which is an essential Part of their Profession, but must take the Words of Druggists, who themselves are sometimes mistaken, and differ about the Names of several Drugs; and which is worse, their trusting to Herb-women, who obtrude almost any thing upon the greatest Part of them; and that those Women do often mistake one Thing for another, sometimes ignorantly, sometimes designedly, is well known to many Physicians, who have seen them sell the Apothecaries Herbs, Roots and Seeds, under other Names than those they do really bear, for many among them cannot distinguish between Ingredients noxious and salutary: So that we have not Patients daily poisoned is rather from the Care of Herb-women than Apothecaries. Another just Cause of Complaint against the Apothecaries are, their old Medicines; for suppose them as faithfully prepared as they can pretend or we desire, yet Length of Time will make some Changes in them, which are not often Improvements: The Syrups grow acid, and Waters full of Mother, Electuaries and Pills dry and deprived of their most active Parts, Powders themselves are not free from this Fate, whose Virtues in Time we find marvelously diminished. But were they to be told of this, you may with as good Success preach to a Wall, for not a Dram of any other Medicine will the Apothecaries part with but for Sale: So that many times they sell their Preparations five or six Years after they were made, and whether their Medicinal Properties are not much impaired, if they have any left, we leave to others to determine. And indeed the Apothecary has many Things in his Shop which are not called for in many Months, yet these must be vended with the rest; all which, when they have lost their Virtues, should they be rejected, it would be much to their Prejudice, and they have a fundamental Practice that no such Thing should be allow'd of: For 'tis much better the Patient should suffer somewhat in his Body than the Apothecary in his Estate; and if he has injured by his bad Physick, perhaps he will take Pity of him, and the next Prescription shall be better prepared; whereby he makes him abundance of Recompence for the Hurt he receiv'd by that which was bad: And he himself makes an Advantage of both, although perhaps if he had consulted the Patient, he would rather have chosen to keep his Head sound than have it broken, that a proper Plaister might be applied for the Cure. This is so notorious a Truth, that all the World, even their best Friends, exclaim against them for it, and 'till they amend this among many other Peccadillo's, it behoves the Patient to take care how seldom he employs them. Another, that the Apothecaries and their Servants are so careless, slovingly and slight in preparing of dispensatory, or prescribed Medicines, that neither the Physicians, or the Diseased, have Reason to repose that Trust in them which they challeng'd as their Due. As for Slovenliness, they may, I confess, plead the old Proverb, *That what the Eyes see not, the Heart rues not.* Indeed of all the rest it may be dispensed with; but should Patients but once behold how their Physick was prepared in some Shops, they would nauseate it: But least I should offend some nice Stomachs, I shall dismiss this Subject, and proceed to another, which is the Carelessness of Apothecaries and their Apprentices; on which I can never reflect without Fear and Indignation, to think what Numbers have been destroy'd and injur'd by such Proceedings: That this is not a groundless Apprehension many Families can witness, and you can converse with few Persons who are not able to give an Account of some such Miscarriages.

Another thing of great Blame with the Apothecaries is, their enhancing the Prices of Medicines so much above what they might in Reason expect; about which the Physician must no ways concern himself, because it has a bad Influence on him, as on the Account of his Patient; though certainly, if the Apothecaries were more modest in the prising of their Physick, the Patient would be more liberal to the Physician: Whereas on the contrary, the Apothecary holds them at such unreasonable Rates, that in most Courses of Physick he gains more than the Doctor, how deservedly let others determine, though in my Opinion, were their Pay proportion'd to their Care and Honesty, I doubt they would gain little besides Shame and Reproaches: But their Bills must be paid without Abatement; and with how much Regret they are discharg'd, I shall refer it to those who have suffered by them. Now several Things contribute to, or are the occasional Causes of this Universal

Grievance. The Physician's Silence, and the Number, Pride, or Covetousness of the Apothecaries, and that Prices are not set upon their Medicines: the Apothecaries being reduc'd into a Company, were at first few; and therefore having full Employment, could afford their Medicines at moderate Prices; but being since that time increased to a great Number, each Person bringing up two or three, or more, that Imployment which was before in a few Hands, became more dispers'd, so that very small Portion thereof falls to the Share of some, and indeed very few of them have more than they can manage. Now the Sick must maintain all these, for although there be no occasion for a sixth Part, yet they must all live handsomely; to supply which Expence, they have no other Way than to exalt the Prices of their Medicines, and still the less they are employ'd, the higher they must prize them, otherwise they could not possibly subsist, unless they became Physicians, and prescribe as well as prepare; to which Practices they are not only propense, but more arrogantly assume, which is no less fatal to their Patients, than by the impudent Prescription of your common Quacksalver, Emperic, or Mountebank.

Now would it not be much better, if it were with us as in some Parts of *Europe*, where the Magistrates of many Cities agree upon a certain Number of Apothecaries, so many as they can apprehend are necessary, all the rest are excluded, and must either seek other Seats, or be content for a small Salary to work under those that are allow'd; their Apothecaries not being permitted to multiply by Apprentices, but one out of the Shop is by the publick Authority appointed to succeed in the Employment. *Hamburgh* has but one, *Stockholm* and *Copenhagen* four or Five, *Paris* (which rivals *London* in its Inhabitants) has but one or two and fifty; they are from the due Regard to the Safety of the People exempted from Offices, either troublesome or profitable, that they may always be inspecting the Preparations, or compounding of the Doses, to prevent the deadly Consequences of sophisticated Medicines, or the fatal Errors of one Composition for another, not easily to be distinguished: They are not permitted to visit the Sick, that they may not be wanting from the Duties of the Shop, or be tempted to gratify themselves as they please for the Trouble, by introducing the Custom of taking too often of the Bolus and Cordials. The Physicians Fees are settled according to the various Conditions and Abilities of the Patient; 'tis not allow'd them to make any Advantage by the arbitrary Rates of Physick, when prepared by themselves, that the Patient and the Bill may not be too much inflam'd by a Profit on that side, not easily to be limited or confined. I would not be suspected to design any Prejudice to the careful and industrious Apothecary, (if such there be) his Business requires the greatest Diligence and Fidelity in selecting the Drugs, and preparing them faithfully according to the Appointment of the Faculty, and in making up the Doses with that just Regard to the Life of the Sick, that all Suspicion of the least Mistake may be prevented, in the Weight and Measure, or the Number of Drops, *&c.* But when the Apothecary deserts his Station, is always abroad, and leaves the compounding Part to his unexperienc'd Apprentice, who cannot avoid sometimes infusing one thing for another, by which Errors many are known to have lost their Lives; when 'tis known that the Prescripts are made up of Medicines bought by Wholesale of the Chymist, and not made up by the Apothecary himself, as is too much the present Practice, and consequently can't be known to be made of all, and best Ingredients, but are suspected, because bought at low Prices; you will doubt whether the Character of an Apothecary can be given to this new, and till lately unknown Employment: When he neglects the Business of his Trade, neither prepares himself the Compositions, nor forms the Doses for them, to be deliver'd at the most urgent Occasions, but daringly undertakes to advise in all Distempers, he becomes an Emperic, and invades a Profession which he cannot be supposed to understand.

And here give me Leave to be serious, in examining their general Practice in all Diseases. Suppose your self to be troubled with any Distemper, it matters not which, for all is one to him you send to; upon his Arrival he feels your Pulse, and with a fix'd Eye upon your Countenance, tells you your Spirits are low, and therefore it's high time for a Cordial; the next Interogatory he puts gravely to you is, When was you at Stool, Sir? if not to Day, he promises to send you a laxative Clyster by and by; and if you complain you have a Looseness, then instead of one laxative, he will send you two healing Clysters: If besides you intimate a Pain in your Stomach, Back and Sides, then, responding to each Pain, you shall have a Stomach Plaister, another for the right Side, another for the left, and one for the Back, and so you are like to have a large Patch and well fortified round the Middle. Now before we go farther, let's compute the Charge of the first Day. There is the Cordial, composed by the Direction of some old dusty Bill on his File, out of two or three musty Waters (especially if it be towards the latter End of the Year, and that his Glasses have been stopt with Corks) *viz.* it may be a Citron, a Borrage and a Baum Water, all very full of Spirits, if River Water may be so accounted; to these is to be added one Ounce of that miraculous Treakle Water, then to be dissolved a Dram of *Confectio Alkermes*, and one Ounce of nauseous Syrup of July-Flowers; this being well shaked in the Vial, you shall spy a great Quantity of Gold swimming in Leaves up and down, for which your Conscience would be burthened should you give him less than Five Shillings; for from the meanest Tradesman he expects, without Abatement, Three and Six pence, the ordinary and general Price of all Cordials, tho' consisting only of Baum Water and half an Ounce of Syrup of July-Flowers. Your Clyster shall be prepared out of two or three Handsful of Mallow Leaves and one Ounce of common Fennil Seeds, boiled in Water to a Pint, which strained, shall be thickned with the common Electuary lenitive, Rape Oil and brown Sugar, and so seasoned with Salt; this shall be convey'd into your Guts by the young Doctor, his Man, through an Engine he commonly carries about with him, and makes him smell so wholsome; for which Piece of Service if you present your Engineer with less than Half a Crown, he will think himself worse dealt with than those who empty your necessary Closets in the Night; the Master places to Account for the Gut-Medicine (though it were no more than Water and Salt) and for the Use of his Man, which he calls Porteridge, Eight Groats. *Item*, For a Stomatick, Hepatick, Splenetick, and a Nephretick Plaister, for each Half a Crown: What the Total of this Day's Physick does amount to you may reckon. The next Afternoon or Evening the Apothecary returns himself to give you a Visit, (for should he appear in the Morning, it would argue he had little to do) and finding, upon Examination, you are rather worse than better, by Reason those Plaisters caused a melting of the gross Humours about the Bowels, and dissolved them into Winds and Vapours, which fuming to the Head, occasion a great Head-ach, Dulness and Drowsiness, and Part of 'em being dispersed through the Guts and Belly, discompose you with a Cholick, a Swelling of your Belly, and an universal Pain or Lassitude over all your Limbs. Thus you see one Day makes Work for another; however, he hath the Wit to assure you, they are Signs of the Operations of Yesterday's Means, beginning to move and dissolve the Humours; which successful Work is to be promoted by a Cordial Apozem, the Repetition of a carminative Clyster, another Cordial to take by Spoonfuls, and because your Sleep has been interrupted by the Unquietness of swelling Humours, he will endeavour to procure you for this next Night a Truce with your Disease, by an Hypnotick Potion that shall occasion Rest: Neither will he give you any other Cause than to imagine him a most careful Man, and so circumspect, that scarce a Symptom shall pass his particular Regard; and therefore to remove your Head-ach by retracting the Humours, or rather, as you are like to discern best, by attracting Humours and Vapours, he will order his young Mercury to apply a Vesicatory to the Nape of your Neck, and with a warm Hand to besmear your Belly and all your Joints with a good comfortable Ointment for to appease your Pains: The Cordial Apozem is a Decoction that shall derive its Virtue from two or three unsavoury Roots, and as many Herbs and Seeds, with a little Syrup of July-Flowers, for three or four Times taking; which because you shall not undervalue by having it brought to you all in one Glass, you shall have it sent you in so many Vials and Draughts, and for every one of them shall be placed Three Shillings to your own Account, which is five Parts more than the Whole stands him in; for the Cordial Potion as much; for the Hypnotick Potion the same Price; for your Carminative Clyster no less; and for the Epispastick Plaister a Shilling: Thus with the Increase of your Disease you may perceive the Increase of your Bill; and therefore it's no improper Observation, That the Apothecaries Practice follow the Course of the Moon. The third Day produces an Addition of new Symptoms, and an Augmentation of the old ones; the Patient stands in need of new Comfort from his Apothecary, who tells him, that Nature begins now to work more strong, and therefore all Things go well (and never ill;) but because Nature requires all possible Assistance from Cordials and small Evacuations, he must expect to have the same Cordials over again, but with the Addition of greater Ingredients, it may be Magistery of Pearl, or Oriental Bezoar in Powder, besides the Repetition of a Clyster, and the renewing of your Plaisters, for the Profit of your Physician, you must be persuaded to accept of a comfortable Electuary for the Stomach, to promote Digestion; of a Collution to wash your Gums to secure you from the Scurvy, serving at the same Time to wash the Slime and Filth from your Tongue; of a Melilot Plaister to apply to the Blister that was drawn the Night fore; of some Spirits of Salt to drop into your Beer at Meals; of three Pills of Ruffi to be swallowed down that Night, and three next Morning, which possibly may pleasure you with three Stools, but are to be computed at two Doses, each at a Shilling; the Spirit of Salt a Crown the Ounce; for the Stomach Electuary as much, for the Clysters as before; for your Cordial in relation to the Pearl and Bezoar, their Weight in Gold, which is Two-pence a Grain, the greatest Cheat of my whole Discourse; for dressing your Blister a Shilling; for the Plaister as formerly. Here I presume that Candour in you, as not to believe me so disingenuous, as to take the Advantage of Apothecaries in producing any other than the best Methods of their Practice, and that which favours the least of their Frauds, for in Comparison with others (though these are very palpable, in regard there is not a valuable Consideration regarded as a *quid pro quo*) they are such as may be judged passable; yet when you are to reflect upon the Total that shall arise on the Arithmetical Progression of Charge of a Fortnights Physick, modestly computed at about Fifteen Shillings a Day, without the Inclusion of what you please to present him for his Care, Trouble, and Attendance, I will not harbour so ill an Opinion of him, or give so rigid a Censure as your self shall upon the following Oration your Clysterpipe Doctor delivers to you with a melancholy Accent, in these Terms: Sir, I have made use of my best Skill and Endeavours, I have been an Apothecary these twenty Years, and upwards, and have seen the best Practice of our best *London* Physicians; my Master was such a one, Mr. ——— one of the ablest Apothecaries of the City; I have given you the best Cordials that can be prescrib'd; 'tis at your Instance I did it, I can do no more, and indeed it is more properly the Work of a Physician; your Case is dangerous, and I think, if you sent for such a one, Dr. —— he is a very pretty Man; if you please I will get him to come down. Now, Sir, how beats your Pulse? The Loss of your Monies your Bills import, give Addition to your Pain, through the Remembrance it is due to one that hath fool'd you out of it, and deserv'd it no other way, than by adding Wings to your gross Humours that before lay dormant, and now fly rampant up and down, raking, and raging; which had you not been Penny wise and Pound foolish, you would have prevented by sending for a Physician, who for the small Merit of a City-Fee (for which you might also have expected two Visits) would have struck at the Root of the Distemper, without tampering at its Symptoms, or Branches, and by Virtue of one Medicine, restor'd you to your former Condition of Health from which you are now so remote, being necessitated, considering your doubtful State, to be at the Charge of a Physician or two, to whom, upon Examination of what hath been done before, the Apothecary shall humbly declare, he hath given you nothing but Cordials; which Word Cordial, he supposes to be a sufficient Protection for his erroneous Practice; and I must tell you, that had his Cordial Method been continu'd in a Fever, or any other acute Distemper, for eight or ten Days, your Heirs would have been particularly obliged to him for giving you a Cordial Remove out of your Possession, and that through Omission of those two great Remedies, Purging and Bleeding, the exact Use whereof, in respect of Time and Quantity, and other Circumstances, can only be determined by accomplish'd Physicians.

I cannot better describe their Unaptness for so great a Work, nor express the great Difficulties that must be conquer'd to deserve the first Character of a compleat Physician, than in the Words of that eminent and learned Physician Dr. *Fuller*; 'It requires (says he) to understand the learned Languages, Natural Philosophy, all the Parts of the Body, and the Animal Oeconomy, the Nature, Causes, Times, Tendencies, Symptoms, Diognosticks, and Prognosticks of Diseases, the Indications of Cure, and contra Indications, the Rules of Errors of living as to the Six Non-naturals; we must have the Skill to judge to whom, for what, when, how much, how often to prescribe Bleeding, Vomiting, Purging, Sweating, and other Evacuations; as also to Opiates, Calybiates, Cortex, and the numberless other Alteratives: We must be very well acquainted with the Virtues, Faults, Preparations, Compositions, and Doses of Vegetables, Animals, Minerals, and all Shop Medicines; and lastly, to compleat all, must be able, upon every emergent Occasion, to write a Bill for a Patient, readily, pertinently, and in Form according to Art. Now to accomplish all this, a Man had need be rightly born, and set out by Nature, with a peculiar Genius, and particular Fitness, and with a strong prevailing Inclination to this Study and Practice above all others.

'He must endeavour with Diligence, Sagacity and Gravity, Integrity, and such a convenient Briskness and Courage as will bear him up, and carry him through Difficulties, without presumptuous Rashness or barbarous Hard-heartedness; and then 'tis necessary he should be a Man of a competent Estate, to answer the great Expence of Education and Expectation; for he must be brought up directly in it from the Beginning of his Studies in the University; he must lay out all his Time and Talents upon Reading, Advising, Observing, Experimenting, Reasoning, Remembering, with an unwearied

Labour of Body and Application of Mind; he must run through Courses of Anatomy, Botany, Chymistry and *Galenick* Pharmacy: And when he hath done all this, cannot handsomely compleat himself, except he see good Variety of others practise, which (by the by) it's probable he will have more Time for than he could wish, before he can get any of his own.'

Now each of those singly will require a great deal of Pains, Expence and Time to be attained; and yet all these and much more that can be in short summed up, ought to be done and in some measure accomplished, before a Man can be rightly and duly qualified even to begin Practice.

And as to Matter of Fact, few (very few, God knows) there have been, or now are, who tho' they spared not for Education or Diligence, ever work themselves up to a tolerable Sufficiency: Nay, *Hippocrates* himself, that great Genius, is not ashamed to confess, in an Epistle to *Democritus*, That though he was now got to Old Age and to the End of Life, yet he was not got to the End of Physick; no, nor was *Æsculapius* neither, the Inventor of it.

By all which, it's undeniably evident, that the Science and Practice of Physick is one of the largest Studies, and most difficult Undertakings in the World; and consequently, not any the best Collection of Prescripts that ever was, will, or can be writ or printed, can alone make a compleat Physician, any more than good Colours and Pencils alone can make a fine Painter. And yet every illiterate Fellow and paltry Gossip that can make shift to patch up a Parcel of pitiful Receipts, have the Impudence and Villainy to venture at it; and in hopes of a good Pig, Goose or Basket of Chickens, shall boldly stake their Skill (forsooth) against Mens Lives, and lose them; and at the same Time scandalize and keep out true Physicians, that might probably save them.

And this leads me to the third Consideration, The great Danger and Damage occasioned by the rash tampering of such as are not educated rightly and qualified for it.

You that enter not by the Door into the Profession, but climb up some other Way, ought to take it into your most serious Thoughts, that Mistakes and Mismanagement in so difficult a Business easily happen; often the Mischiefs occasioned thereby are impossible to be retrieved; and being upon the Body, perhaps Mind of Man, sometimes produce such undoing Misery, such deplorable Ruin, as would make even an Heart of Stone break and bleed, and Death to think of it. Suppose one should lose his Limbs or Health, and live unhappily in Pain, Sick or Bedrid all his Days through your improper Applications or ignorant Omissions; Would it not turn your very Bowels within you, and make you wish a thousand times you had never been that unadvis'd Busie-body to act thus foolishly and unfortunately?

But put the Case again: You behold a dead Man (which to me is the most lamentable of all lamentable Spectacles Upon Earth) I say, put Case a poor dead Man were laid before your Eyes, that your Heart tells you might probably have lived many a fair Year, had it not been for your physicking of him: Such a Sight, such a Thought, (if you have the least Humanity left) cannot fail to pierce your very Soul; and ever after the Remembrance, yea, the evil Conscience of it must haunt you and give you Horror and Terror, and a sort of Hell to your dying Hour.

Perhaps it may be an only and hopeful Son, in whose Life his aged Parents Lives were bound up; and they die too, or linger out a miserable Life in Sorrow and Anguish worse than Death.

Perhaps the good Father of a many little Orphans, who being poor and now helpless, must pitiously perish, or being fallen into bad Hands, and cheated of what was left them, may suffer Poverty, Contempt, Injury and Misery all their Life long.

Perhaps a Wife, who might have brought forth an useful eminent Man, a Hero of his Generation, and the Head of splendid Families; and so the Mischief you do may fall upon not only the present but future Ages.

But Possibilities and putting of Cases are endless, the Upshot of all this, if you take upon you to cure the Sick, and be not licensed and otherwise qualified for it, if you presumptuously thrust in your self, and bar out another that is authorized and able, though no ill Event chance thereupon, yet well it might, and was likely to do so for all you; and therefore good Providence that protected your Patient, and fenced off the Evils, is alone to be thanked, and you nevertheless to be blamed.

But if Death ensue your arrogant Intermeddling and pernicious Quackery, be assured of it, 'tis a sort of Murder in the Court of Conscience, and probably will be adjudged so in the last Great Court.

This is not my private Opinion only, but the Judgment and Decision of the Legislature of our Land; for the *Present State of* England tells us, That by the Law of *England*, if one who is no Physician or Surgeon, and not expresly allow'd to practise, shall take upon him a Cure, and his Patient die under his Hands, this is Felony in the Person presuming so to do.

'Tis not enough for you to say, If I can do no Good, I'll do no Hurt, (which you may as well invert, and say, If I do no Hurt I'll do no Good) no, you interlope, you injure the Faculty, you discourage Education, you keep out better Advice, you trifle with Mens Lives, you lose the golden Opportunity, you prolong the Case 'till it gets head, and grows incurable and mortal, or else extremely hazardous and almost helpless; and this is doing Hurt with a Vengeance.

To bring this home to you, and make it more plain. If an House be on Fire, and you come and pretend to put it out your self, and absolutely keep off others, and then fling in Dust instead of Water, and so the Flame gets Mastery; in this Case, though you did not directly intend any positive Hurt, though you did not actually pour in Oil, nor stir and blow up the Coals; yet forasmuch as you would needs be an Undertaker, and could not extinguish it your self, and suffered not others, used to and skill'd in the Business, who coming with Water and proper Engines, might have done it, you are really and truly the Cause of it being burnt.

Think not to excuse your self by pretending you did it out of Charity, and meant well, though it fell out ill; no, no, be it known to you, such a Charity as did not appertain to you, and proved murderous, was unpardonable Presumption, and therefore will not cover the multitude of Sins.

If you are not sufficient for those Things, you'll do well and wisely to desist from this difficult and dangerous Practice, and fall into such a Trade of Life as you well understand and rightly can manage. And then like the Men who used curious Arts (*Acts* xix. 19.) you may burn all your Receipt-Books; so shall you keep your Innocence, save your Conscience, secure your Quiet, and yet reserve Room enough to exercise your Charity.

For if at any Time your Heart move you to pity and succour a poor sick Neighbour that can't pay for Advice, there will be no Necessity that you should try your Skill upon him, 'till you mischief or murder him by way of Charity. Do but you send him a Physician, Medicines and Necessaries without Hope of Requital; and trust me, that will be an handsome Assistance, most nobly becoming a generous Mind and a charitable Man.

Now that not one of our Apothecaries, or indeed very few of our modern Traders in Physick, have these requisite Endowments, I shall leave it to any considerate Person to judge of; and how far they stretch beyond their Knowledge, we have a many miserable Objects in our daily View, woful Instances of their great Rashness, Folly and Ignorance.

That the Profession has sunk into the Craft of deceiving, and amusing, and making Profit by new Medicines, or useless Preparations brought into fashion, and highly esteem'd, as long as the Mode of crying them up shall last, and the Fallacy which imposes them can support it, the unhappy People suffer themselves to be deluded, and cheated of their Lives, and their Money. The Rich please themselves that they can purchase the Alexipharmic, which has Power to controul the Disease, and have not any Doubt within themselves, that by the often Use, their Lives become almost immortal; they look down with some small Pity on the Vulgar, who they think must die before them, being not able to pay the Ransom. They please themselves, because Health and Life are of the highest Demands for these Rarities peculiar to them. The Gentlemen of both the higher and lower Faculty have not been wanting to make use of the Credulity and Weakness of the richer Patients; and I shall now lay open to your great Surprize, that the most despicable and useless Stuff have been brought into the highest Esteem to be rely'd on in the most difficult and dangerous Distempers.

And *First*, of the *Bezoar*-Stone, an obvious Instance of our *English* Practice, from whence you may concur with the Physicians abroad, with what Skill, and Art, and Integrity the Profession continues to be practised here.

Bezoar (which has neither Smell nor Taste, and upon taking into the Stomach gives no Sensation perceivable) has held its Name and Reputation almost sacred with us, though exploded long since in almost all Parts of *Europe*. The *French* are well convinced that they have been impos'd upon by the trading Physicians returning from the *Indies*, to take off the pretty Trifle at a very great Price; they had made it to be admired, by asserting that it was able to encounter Poisons, that no malignant Distempers were able to resist its soveraign Virtues; but their overdoing, spoilt their Market, the more curious and wiser Part of the Nation discerning the Abuse, had the Opportunity of promoting the Experiment, which they procured by the King's Command, two Criminals who had Poison given them, with Promise of Life, if *Bezoar* could procure their Pardon. They lost their Lives, and the Physicians and the Stone their Reputations. The greatest and most learned abroad have freely own'd that they have been deceiv'd by it, but their Patients much more, who had used it without Success, and any observable Effect.

Doctor *Pauli* tells you, he has left the Use of it many Years, and had given to better Purpose, the more powerful and certain Cordials taken from Plants; and supports his Opinion with the Suffrages of *Casper*, *Bauhinus*, *Casp. Hofmanus*, *Rectius*, *Fabriciùs*; The learned and judicious *Deemoebreck* in his Treatise of the Pestilence, declares he had no Regard to it, that he gave it often *absque ullo fructu, movebat aliquo modo exiguum duntaxit sudorem*. It did, says he, no good to those who used it; scarcely mov'd so much as a little Sweat: It was of the best Parcel chosen of any coming from the *Indies*, or ever was sent to *Europe*, but gave them not the least Relief, though they had promised themselves the greatest from it: To confirm his Opinion that it is worth nothing, he produces the Opinion of *Hercules Saxonias*, and *Crato* Physician to three Emperors, and refers you to many others. Doctor *Patin*, late Royal Professor of Physick in *Paris*, decides the Pretences to its being of any kind of Use: He says it neither stirs the Blood, nor puts the Spirits in any Motion; besides, some of the above-nam'd Physicians, he appeals to the Judgment of many others, and his own Experience of more than thirty Years. The lately corrected *Leewarden*'s Dispensatory leaves it out of their *Gascoins Powder*, condemning it as a useless and frivolous Ingredient.

Bontius tells you, that if we must give Stones, we ought to put a greater Value upon those cut out of the Bladders of Man, a more noble Creature, fed with Meat of the highest Nourishment, and his Spirits warm'd with Wine, than that of a Goat starving upon the Mountains. He assures you that he has given the *Bezoar*, from the Gall or the Bladder, with better Effect than he ever observ'd of those from the *Indies*. The Physicians who first began the Amusement and Cheat, made themselves ridiculous by dreading to give for a Dose more than five, or six, or seven Grains: You may take forty or fifty with no other Advantage or Alteration than your Imagination shall raise; and with the same Effect, ten times as much more. It may, with modern Observers, pass for a Sweater, and a Cordial, when they have given it with good Cordials, and Sweaters, but the most visible Operation it has, is seen when the Bill is paid. Our Physicians in their private Conversations, talk of it as a thing altogether worthless; but because the People are willing to be cheated with *Bezoar* and *Pearl*, they dare not entertain a Thought of undeceiving them, fearing the Consequence to their own Disadvantage: And I pray with what Art can the high Rate of Medicines be maintain'd, if the World could not be amused with the Imagination of being kept alive in all the Distempers, by the Force of these two?

Pearl is a Disease in a Shell-Fish, as *Bezoar* is in the *Quadruped*: They are very different in Shape and Bulk, the whitest and most glittering are most in Esteem; the sickly Fancy conceits it will revive the Blood as it pleases the Eye; and that it will brisk up the Spirits and Mind, when it reflects on its being dear and fashionable. But this has been despis'd by the honest Physicians, who prescribe for the Cure of their Patients. The famous *Plater*, after the Experience of a many Years Practice, rejects the pretended Virtues of Pearl, or Metals, which have no Taste or Smell, to give the least Pretence to rank them with the Vegetable Alexipharmicks.

Most of our Writers are of his Sentiment, and give it only a common Place with the others usually prescrib'd in the Heart-burning, or windy sour Humour offending the upper Orifice of the Stomach: But the Shell of the Fish that breeds them, pretends to, and is allow'd by all our best Authors to have the same Virtues. Nature has been very liberal in this Sort of *Alkali*; all the Shell-fish, all the Claws of Crabs, or the Tips, if you please to value them most, the two Stones of the Craw-fish, and the Shells of Eggs are directed frequently with the Pearl: The two Corals, *&c.* and the numerous Earths of the absorbing Kind, the Chalk, the Marles, are judged by many preferable to it, or are used with the same Success: So that we have the greatest Reason to believe, that the debauched Practice of the *English* Preservers of Health have made use of it, with Design to extract Sums out of the Purse, rather than of making the Crasis of the Blood better, or the Spirits more vivacious; and if you have Oyster-Shells or Crabs-Eyes in its Stead, which are generally made use of under that Name, they will have the same, if not a better Effect.

Gold is by our Chymical Writers stil'd the Sun, and the King of Metals. The Kings and Princes of the last Age were amus'd and defrauded, their Lives made less durable than their Subjects, who were beneath the Use of Gold; the Chicken they eat had the Happiness to be fed with it, that they might extract the Sulphur and prepare it by their Circulation, and volatize it for their Use. But the Physicians were contented to collect all the Gold which past unaltered and undiminished thro' the Poultry, into their Pockets. This, with many other Artifices of this Stamp, are by many laid aside, because the Publick begin to be sensible that the Gold, as the *Bezoar* and the Pearl, were of more Cordial Virtue to the Adviser and Confederates than to the Subject of their Care and Attendance.

The *Aurum potabile* is sometime the Entertainment of Conversation, when the poor Alcymists or their vain Pretensions are considered; there being no Humour in any Animal which can alter or dissolve it, no Effect or Operation can be expected from it, it deludes the Eye and Fancy in the Cordial Waters, and on the Bolus and Electuaries, but must pass away sooner or later as it adheres more or less to the Stomach or Bowels, without acting or being acted on in any Part of the Body; the Pills, either purgative or cordial, are as often dismist entire, having been covered with Leaf-Gold, which is able, though thin, to dismiss the most subtil and penetrating Parts of all Humours. The Value of the Leaf is not worth your Enquiry, the Book being sold at a low Price. The Fulminating Powder is a rough violent Medicine, and has been lately neglected, and given Place to others more useful and less dangerous.

Silver and Lunar Pills are as vile and disregardless as Gold, when they are considered with relation to the Cure of Diseases.

The precious Stones have constantly been put into the old Receipts by that Sort of Writers who prescribe every Medicine very faithfully, and design to please and amuse the Readers with the Bulk and Length of the Prescription; but they have been neglected by the practical Authors, who had the Trouble of considering, that no Manner of Vertue could be expected from so hard and therefore impenetrable Bodies; as the Diamond, Ruby, Hyacinth, the Sapphire, the Smargad and Topaz, *&c.* who are not capable of a Dissolution, and of altering or acting upon the Fluids, and as it is most certain that many very cheap Medicines have greater and more observable Effects, it's ridiculous to give a hard gritty Powder, which may for many Reasons corrode and offend the Stomach and Bowels in their Passage.

Among the many Foreign Vegetables imported here, I must take Notice of Sarsaparilla, as it has had the Preference before many others, especially of our own Growth, in many difficult and chronical Cases, will have obtain'd its Credit and Reputation by being in good Company, and by being prescrib'd with the cheapest Drugs, but of the greatest Virtues, *viz.* Guiacum, Sasaphras, China, and the Seeds of many most useful Plants. If it has been by it self beneficial, in the Practice of the *West-Indies*, it has lost its Qualities in the Passage into the colder Climates, being a soft and thin Root, it may evaporate and exhale its most active Parts; many of the late Writers have given this Judgment of it, that it is *nullius Saporis vel Odoris*, of no Smell or Taste.

The Physicians have not yet done, but contrive to thrust into the Stomachs of their Patients, not only the most loathsome, but the Parts of Animals, which after their Death, are void of all Spirits or Oils, and are a dry and unactive Earth.

Of the first Sort, Mummy claims the Precedence; this has had the Honour to be worn in the Bosom next to the Heart, by the Kings and Princes, and all those who could then bear the Price the last Age in all the Courts of *Europe*; 'twas presented with the greatest Assurance, that it was able to preserve from the most deadly Infections, and that the Heart was secured by it from all the Kinds of Malignity: They expected long Life from the decay'd, or dead, Spices, and Balsams, and Gums, and the Piece of the dead Body of an *Egyptian* Prince, or of a Slave preferred by him: If taken inwardly, it was avow'd to be able to dissolve the Blood coagulated, to give new Life and Motion to all the Spirits. The dry'd Hearts of many Animals, the Livers, the Spleens burnt to a Powder; the Skins of the Stomachs, or Guts of Cocks, and Worms, and the dry'd Lungs of Foxes, ought to be rejected as loathsome and offensive without any Qualities to amend, by the Expectation of any Advantage.

The Powder of Vipers by it self, and in the Troches, will deserve a more strict Examination, because it is not only depended on in many Chronical Diseases, but the Life of the Patient in the Acute and Pestilential is betray'd and lost, if it has no alexiterial Powers to expel the Malignity, or support the natural Vigour. But as the Flesh of all Animals, and Fish, when dry'd, have exhal'd the Volatile Spirits with the Moisture, and nothing remains but the Skins and Fibres, and are capable of giving very little Nourishment to the Blood, and are very difficult to be dissolv'd, or digested in the Stomach: You may conclude, by trying when in Health, if Vipers will support your Strength, or if eating of the Flesh in all the Kinds of Cookery, will please the Palate more than the common Food, what you may hope from the dry Powder, or the Cake of it with Salt and Meal, (and the Troches of Vipers are no more) when your Fever calls for the best Alexipharmick. You may to this compare the Skulls of dead Men, now presum'd to command the Epilepsies, and other violent Diseases, if the Skull has been long in Powder, or has long surviv'd the Criminal, the Spirits distill'd from it, are not stronger than those from the Horn of a Stag, or the Spirits of Urin by it self, or from Sal Armoniack: the

Shell of the Head preserves the Brains, and the Powder shall not fail to preserve the Spirits of all the Brains which can be perswaded to use it.

What can you think will be the Success, from the Use of the Nest of the Swallow, or the Cast off Skin of a Serpent; your Thoughts will naturally reflect on the perfidious Fourbery of making great Gain from the Bubbles put on the Sick, or the vile Negligence of the rest who have suffer'd the fatal Amusements to be at last confirm'd by Custom.

After these it may seem needless to speak of the gainful Industry, which has brought the Horns of the Elk, the Bufalo, Rhinoceros, and of the Unicorn's Horn, which is no other than the Bone of a Fish, and has been thought sufficient alone to expel all Poisons; or the Hoofs of the Elk and the Ounce, or the Bone of the Hart of a Stag, the Effect of his old Age; or the Jaw-bones of the Pyke, *&c.* or the Ancle-bones of the Hares and Boars, *&c.* with the Eagle-Stone, and those for the Cramp, and Convulsions, and Cholicks, the great Assistance from your Amulets, and abounding Nostrums, cannot sufficiently be derided.

Of the simple distill'd Waters, one hundred and fifty are appointed to be made, the greatest Part of them are not now prepar'd; and indeed they are found of no Use, but to increase the Bulk of the Julep, with the hot and compound Waters; the Milk Water is now order'd for that Design, and because as much Money can be procur'd from it, as from all the vast Variety of the other, this in the usual Practice almost supplies the Place of all the rest. You may run over the vast Number of the *Galenical* Preparations and Compositions, as they are improperly stiled; they are almost seven hundred, to be kept till they be corrupt, and be viewed as the old rusty and rotten Weapons of an ancient Armory; they are now reduc'd to, and the Shop is supposed to be made up with about One hundred and fifty: But if the insipid Simple Waters, and the fiery ungrateful Compound Waters shall be thrown aside, and the Simple Milk Water, with five or six Cordial Tinctures, shall be kept for Use, and the other Tincture appointed by the Physician, with respect to the Circumstances of the Patient: If only three or four Syrups and Conserves, and Powders, and Pills, and Oils, and Ointments, and Plaisters in that Number, in Imitation of the Prudence and Integrity of the Foreign Physicians who have contracted their Dispensatories, shall be order'd, in the most rational, and efficacious Forms, to receive the Addition of all the natural Powders, Balsams, Gums, or the Chymical Medicines, the Apothecary will have his Trouble very much lessened, and with less Expence; the Patient will have his Disease much sooner cured, and his Life much better preserved.

By this time we presume the Reader is convinc'd, that private Interest too often influences many of our Modern Physicians, and makes them prescribe such Medicines as tend most to the Apothecaries Gain, because the People give the Apothecary Power of appointing the Physician; we have shewn that those costly pretended Medicines, which so much raise the Sum in the Bill, have no real Virtue; that the greatest Part of the most senative grow in our own Gardens; that if some few are fetch'd from foreign Parts, they are used in so small Quantities, that the Doses are of the lowest Price: And consequently you will very plainly see, that the long and high charg'd Bill after a Fit of Sickness, is more the Effect of the Collusion betwixt the Doctor and Apothecary, together with your own Folly of desiring of it, than either the Prices of the Medicine, or the Necessity of so many Doses.

I dare say, my Reader now thinks it high time to take Care of himself, to believe that the seldomer the Physician or Apothecary are employ'd, the less Risque he runs in his Health or Fortune, that he is not upon every slight Indisposition, or ordinary Sickness to call upon their Help, whereby very often the Remedy proves worse than the Disease; that your Constitution will endeavour to preserve it self, and will effect it in most of the common Distempers, but with ill Medicines those will become dangerous, and will be made every Day more malignant. Take the Counsel of your most observing and experienced Friend, who has no Byass to divert him from the only Care of your Health; but avoid the Emperick, who will, instead of procuring the Ease of your Thoughts and Repose, and prescribing the Rules of your Diet, and permitting Nature to subdue the Disease, affright you with the greatest Danger, disturb you, and fill your Chamber, or both, with the inflaming and pernicious Cordials, the Bolus's and Draughts, till he has cured his own Distemper by the Number of Articles he shall enter into the Bill.

That it is in the Power of every Man to become his own Physician, who needs no other Helps of supporting a good, and correcting a bad Constitution, than by observing a sober and regular Life; there is nothing more certain, than that Custom becomes a second Nature, and has a great Influence upon our Bodies, and has too often more Power over the Mind than Reason it self?

The honestest Man alive, in keeping Company with Libertines, by degrees forgets the Maxims of Probity he before was used to, and naturally falls into those Vices with his Companions; and if he be so happy as to acquit himself, and to meet with better Company, then Virtue reassumes its first Lustre, and will triumph in its Turn, and he insensibly regains the Wisdom that he had abandoned.

In a Word, all the Alterations that we perceive in the Temper, Carriage, and Manners of most Men, have scarce any other Foundation, but the Force and Prevalency of Custom.

'Tis an Unhappiness in which the Men of this Age are fall'n, that Variety of Dishes is now the Fashion, and become so far preferable to Frugality; and yet the one is the Product of Temperance, whilst Pride and unrestrain'd Appetite is the Parent of the other.

Notwithstanding the Difference of their Origin, yet Prodigality is at present stiled Magnificence, Generosity and Grandeur, and is commonly esteem'd of in the World, whilst Frugality passes for Avarice and Sordidness in the Eyes and Acceptation of most Men: Here is a visible Error which Custom and Habit have established.

The Error has so far seduc'd us, that it has prevail'd upon us, to renounce a frugal Way of living, though taught us by Nature, even from the first Age of the World, as being that which would prolong our Days, and has cast us into those Excesses, which serve only to abridge the Number of them. We become old before we have been able to taste the Pleasures of being young; and the time which ought to be the Summer of our Lives, is often the beginning of their Winter, we soon perceive our Strength to fail, and Weakness to come on apace, and decline even before we come to Perfection.

On the contrary, Sobriety maintains us in the natural State wherein we ought to be. Our Youth is lasting, our Manhood attended with a Vigour that does not begin to decay 'till after a many Years. A whole Century must be run out before Wrinkles can be form'd on the Face, or Grey-hairs grow on the Head: This is so true, that when Men were not addicted to Voluptuousness, they had more Strength and Vivacity at Fourscore, than we have at present at Forty.

It cannot indeed be expected, that every Man should tie himself strictly to the Observations of the same Rules in his Diet, since the Variety of Climates, Constitution, Age, and other Circumstances may admit of Variations. But this we may assert as a reasonable, general, and undeniable Maxim, founded upon Reason and the Nature of Things; that for the Preservation of Health and prolonging a Man's Life, it is necessary that he eat and drink no more than is sufficient to support his natural Constitution; and on the contrary, whatsoever he eats and drinks beyond, that is superfluous, and tends to the feeding of the corrupt and vicious Humours, which will at last, though they may be stifled for a Time, break out into a Flame and burn the Man quite down, or else leave him like a ruinated or shattered Building.

This general Maxim which we have laid down, will hold good with respect to Men of all Ages and Constitutions, and under whatsoever Climate they live, if they have but the Courage to make a due Application of it, and to lay a Restraint upon their unreasonable Appetites.

After all, we will not, we dare not warrant, that the most strict and sober Life will secure a Man from all Diseases, or prolong his Days to the greatest old Age. Natural Infirmities and Weaknesses, which a Man brings along with him into the World, which he deriv'd from his Parents and could not avoid, may make him sickly and unhealthful, notwithstanding all his Care and Precaution: And outward Accidents (from which no Man is free) may cut off the Thread of Life before it is half spun out. There is no fencing against the latter of those, but as to the former, a Man may in some Measure correct and amend them by a sober and regular Life. In fine, let a Man's Life be longer or shorter, yet Sobriety and Temperance renders it pleasant and delightful. One that is sober, though he lives but thirty or forty Years, yet lives long, and enjoys all his Days, having a free and clear Use of all his Faculties; whilst the Man that gives himself to Excess, and lays no Restraint to his Appetites, though he prolongs his Life to Threescore or Fourscore Years (which is next to a Miracle) yet is his Life but one continu'd doseing Slumber, his Head being always full of Fumes, the Pores of his Soul cloudy and dark, the Organs of his Body weak and worn out, and very unfit to discharge the proper Offices of a rational Creature. And indeed Reason, if we hearken to it, will tell us, that a good Regimen is necessary for the prolonging our Days, and that it consists in two Things, first in takeing Care of the Quality, and secondly of the Quantity, so as to eat and drink nothing that offends the Stomach, nor any more than we can easily digest.

And in this, Experience ought to be our Guide in those two Principles, when we arrive to Forty, Fifty, or Sixty Years of Age. He who puts in Practice that Knowledge which he has of what is good for him, and goes on in a frugal Way of Living, keeps the Humours in a just Temperature, and prevents them from being altered, though he suffer Heat and Cold, though he be fatigued, though his Sleep be broke, provided there be no Excess in any of them. This being so, what an Obligation does Man lie under of living soberly, and ought he not to free himself from the Fears of sinking under the least Intemperature of the Air, and under the least Fatigue, which makes us sick upon every slight Occasion?

'Tis true, the most sober Man may sometimes be indisposed, when they are unavoidably obliged to transgress the Rule which they have been used to observe; but then they are certain, their Indisposition will not last above two or three Days at most, nor can they fall into a Fever: Weariness and Faintness are easily remedied by Rest and good Diet.

There are some who feed high, and maintain, that whatsoever they eat is so little a Disturbance to them, that they cannot perceive in what Part of the Body the Stomach lies; but I averr, they do not speak as they think, nor is it natural? 'Tis impossible that any created Being should be of so perfect a Composition, as that neither Heat nor Cold, Dry nor Moist should have any Influence over it, and that the Variety of Food which they make use of, of different Qualities, should be equally agreeable to them. Those Men cannot but acknowledge, that they are sometimes out of Order; if it is not owing to a sensible Indigestion, yet they are troubled with Head-achs, Want of Sleep, and Fevers, of which they are cured by a Diet, and taking such Medicines as are proper for Evacuations. It is therefore certain, that their Distempers proceed from Repletion, or from their having eat or drank something which did not agree with their Stomachs.

Most old People excuse their high Feeding by saying, that it is necessary to eat a great deal, to keep up their natural Heat, which diminishes proportionably as they grow into Years; and to create an Appetite, 'tis necessary to find out proper Sauces, and to eat whatsoever they have a Fancy for, and that without thus humouring their Palates, they would be soon in their Graves.

To this I reply: That Nature, for the Preservation of a Man in Years, has so composed him, that he may live with a little Food; that his Stomach cannot digest a great Quantity, and that he has no need of being afraid of dying for want of eating; since when he is sick, he is forced to have recourse to a regular Sort of Diet, which is the first and main Thing prescrib'd him by his Physician, that if this Remedy is of such Efficacy to snatch us out of the Arms of Death, 'tis a Mistake to suppose that a Man may not by eating a little more than he does when he is sick, live a long Time without ever being sick.

Others had rather be disturb'd twice or thrice a Year with the Gout, the Sciatica, and their Epidemical Distempers, than to be always put to the Torment and Mortification of laying a Restraint upon their Appetites, being sure, that when they are indisposed, a regular Diet will be an infallible Remedy and Cure. But let them be informed by me, that as they grow up in Years their natural Heat abates; that as regular Diet, despised as a Precaution, and only look'd upon as Physick, cannot always have the same Effect nor Force, to draw off the Crudities, nor repair the Disorders that are caused by Repletion; and lastly, that they run the Hazard of being cheated by their Hope and by their Intemperance.

Others say, That it is more eligible to feed high and enjoy themselves, though a Man live the less while. It is no surprizing Matter that Fools and Mad-men should contemn and despise Life; the World will be no Loser whenever they go out of it; but 'tis a considerable Loss, when wise, virtuous, and holy Men drop into the Grave, who might have done more Honour to their Country and to themselves.

In Youth this Excess is more frequent; necessary therefore it is to moderate his Apetite; for if the Stomach be stretch'd beyond its due Extent, it will require to be fill'd, but never well digest what it receives. Besides, it is much better to prevent Diseases, by Temperance, Sobriety, Chastity, and Exercise, than cure them by Physick.

Quid enim se Medicis dederit, seipsum sibi eripit. Summa Medicinarum ad sanitatem corporis & animæ, abstinentiæ est. He that lives abstemiously, or but temperately, need not study the Wholesomeness of his Meat, nor the Pleasantness of that Sawce, the Moments and Punctillio's of Air, Heat, Cold, Exercise, Lodging, Diet; nor is critical in Cookery or in his Liquors, but takes thankfully what God gives him. Especially, let all young Men forbear Wines and Strong Drinks, as well as spiced and hot Meats; for they introduce a preternatural Heat in the Body, and at least hinder and obstruct, if not at length exhaust the natural.

But if overtaken by Excess, (it's difficult to be always upon our Guard) the last Remedy is vomiting, or fasting it out, neither go to bed on a full Stomach; let Physick be always the last Remedy, that Nature may not trust to it; for though a sick Man leaves all for Nature to do, he hazards much; but when he leaves all for the Doctor to do, he hazards more: And since there is a Hazard both ways, I would sooner rely upon Nature; for this at least we may be sure of, that she is as honest as she can, and that she does not find the Account in prolonging the Disease.

Others there are, who perceiving themselves to grow old, tho' their Stomach be less capable of digesting well every day less than another, yet will not upon that Account abate any thing of their Diet; they only abridge themselves in the Number of their Meals; and because they find two or three Meals a Day is troublesome, they think their Health is sufficiently provided for, by making only one Meal; that so the time between one Repast and another, may (as they say) facilitate the Digestion of those Aliments which they might have taken at twice: For this Reason they eat as much at one Meal, that their Stomach is over-charged and out of Order, and converts the Superfluities of its Nourishment into bad Humours, which engender Diseases and Death.

I never knew a Man live long by this Conduct. These Men would doubtless have prolong'd their Days, had they abridg'd the Quantity of their ordinary Food proportionally as they grew in Years; and had they eat a great deal less a little oftner.

Some again are of Opinion, that Sobriety may indeed preserve a Man in Health, but does not prolong his Life. To this we say, that there have been Persons in past Ages, who have prolong'd their Lives by this Means; and some there are at present who still do it; for as Infirmities contracted by Repletion shorten our Days, a Man of an ordinary Reach may perceive, that if he desires to live long, it is better to be well than sick, and that consequently Temperance contributes more to long Life, than excessive Feeding.

Whatsoever Sensualists may say, Temperance is of infinite Benefit to Mankind: To it he owes his Preservation; it banishes from his Mind the dismal Apprehensions of dying; 'tis by its Means he becomes wise, and arrives to an Age wherein Reason and Experience furnish him with Assistance to free himself from the Tyranny of his Passions, which have lorded it over him for almost the whole Course of his Life.

A very notable Instance of this we have in the Life of *Lewis Cornaro*, a noble *Venetian*, who though of a weakly Constitution, increas'd by a voluptuous Life, yet at the Age of thirty five or forty Years, he was resolv'd to practice in all the Rules of Sobriety and Temperance, and to withdraw from those Excesses that had brought upon him those usual Ills the Gout and the Cholick, fatal Attendants to an indolent and luxurious Life, and which reduc'd him to so low a State, that his Recovery was despair'd of by the wisest Physician: And here he tells you that he was born very cholerick and hasty, and flew out into a Passion for the least Trifle, that he huffed all Mankind, and was so intolerable, that a great many Persons of Repute avoided his Company: He apprehended the Injury which he did to himself, he knew that Anger is a real Frenzy, that it disturbs our Judgment, that it transports us beyond our selves, and that the Difference between a passionate and a mad Man is only this, that the latter has lost his Reason, and the former is only depriv'd of it by fits. A sober Life cured him of his Frenzy; by its Assistance he became so moderate, and so much a Master of his Passions, that no body could perceive it was born with him.

How great and valuable must Temperance then be, which carries that soveraign Aid, and can relieve the Passions of the Mind, and not only to expel the bad Humours of the Body, but also to restore it to a due Tone, and a full State of Health.

Now let any one upon a serious Reflection consider which is most eligible, a sober and regular, or an intemperate, and disorderly Course of Life: This is certain, that if all Men would live regularly and frugally, there would be so few sick Persons, that there would hardly be any Occasion for Remedies,

> *Si tibi deficiant Medici, Medici tibi fiant.*
> *Hæc tria, Mens læta, requies moderata dieta.*
>
> *The best and safest Physician is Doctor Diet,*
> *Doctor Merryman, and Doctor Quiet.*

every one would become his own Physician, and would be convinced that he never met with a better.

It would be to little Purpose to study the Constitution of other Men; every one, if he would but apply himself to it, would always be better acquainted with his own than that of another; every one would be capable of making those Experiments for himself which another could not do for him, and would be the best Judge of the Strength of his own Stomach, and of the

Food which is agreeable thereto; for in one Word, 'tis next to impossible to know exactly the Constitution of another, their Constitutions being as different as their Complexions.

Since no Man therefore can have a better Physician than himself, nor a more soveraign Antidote than a Regimen, that is to study his own Constitution, and to regulate his Life according to the Rules of right Reason.

I own, indeed, the disinterested Physician may be some time necessary, since there are some Distempers, which all human Prudence cannot provide against, there happen some unavoidable Accidents which seize us after such a Manner, as to deprive our Judgment of the Liberty it ought to have to be a Comfort to us; it may then be a Mistake wholly to rely upon Nature, it must be assisted, and Recourse must be had to some one or another for it; and in this we have much the Advantage of the irregular Man, his Vices having heaped Fewel to the Distemper; but on the contrary, by a regular Course of Life, the very Cause is not to be found, and the Disease retreats from you.

And here the fam'd *Cornaro*, who being at Seventy Years of Age, had another Experiment of the Usefulness of a Regimen, and 'twas this; A Business of extraordinary Consequence drawing him into the Country, and being in the Coach, the Horses ran away with him, and was overthrown, and dragg'd a long away before they could stay the Horses; they took him out of the Coach with his Head broke, a Leg and Arm out of joint, and in a Word, in a very lamentable Condition. As soon as they brought him Home again, they sent for the Physicians, who did not expect he should live three Days to an end: However, they resolv'd upon letting of him Blood, to prevent the coming of a Fever, which usually happens upon such Cases. He was so confident that the regular Life which he had led, had prevented the contracting of any ill Humours, of which he might be afraid, that he rejected their Prescription, and ordered them to dress his Head, to set his Leg and Arm, and to rub him with some Specifick Oils proper for Bruises, and without any other Remedies he was soon cured, to the Amazement of the Physicians and of all those that knew him. From hence he did infer, that a regular Life is an excellent Preservative against all natural Ills; and that Intemperance produces quite contrary Effects.

What a Difference then between a sober and an intemperate Life? the one shortens and the other prolongs our Days, and makes us enjoy a perfect Health, and with *Juvenal*, *Mens sana in Corpore sano.* I cannot understand how it comes to pass, that so many People, otherwise prudent and rational, cannot resolve upon laying a Restraint upon their insatiable Appetites at fifty or sixty Years of Age, or at least when they begin to feel the Infirmities of old Age coming upon them they might rid themselves of them by a strict Diet and a due Regimen.

I do not wonder so much that young People are so hardly brought to such a Resolution; they are not capable enough of reflecting; and their Judgment is not solid enough to resist the Charms of Sense: But at Fifty a Man ought to be govern'd by his Reason, which would convince us if we would hearken to it, that to gratify all our Appetites without any Rule or Measure, is the Way to become infirm and die young. Nor does the Pleasure of Taste last long, it hardly begins but 'tis gone and past; the more one eats, the more one may, and the Distempers which it brings along with it, last us to our Graves.

Now should not a sober Man be very well satisfied when he is at Table, upon the Assurance, that as often as he rises from it, what he eats will do him no harm: Who then would not perfectly enjoy the Pleasures of this mortal Life so perfectly? Who will not court and win Sobriety, which is so grateful to God, as being the Guardian to Virtue, and irreconcileable Enemy to Vice.

Surely the Example of this wise and good Man deserves our Imitation, that since old Age may be made so useful and pleasant to Men, I should have fail'd in Point of Charity to inform Mankind by what Methods they might prolong their Days.

A great Assistant to that of Sobriety, and which is highly conducive to the Preservation of the whole Man, is to renew with us that habitual and beneficial Custom of the Antients in promoting *Exercise*, as one great Instrument to the Conservation of Health, and which no one can deny who has given himself the Experience of a Trial.

That it promotes the Digestion, raises the Spirits, refreshes the Mind, and that it strengthens and relieves the whole Man, is scarce disputed by any; but that it should prove curative in some particular Distempers, and that too when scarce any thing else will prevail, seems to obtain little Credit with most People, who though they will give the Physician the hearing when he recommends the Use of Rideing, or any other Sort of Exercise, yet at the Bottom, look upon it as a forlorn Method, and rather the Effects of his Inability to relieve them, than a Belief that there is any great Matter in what he advises: Thus by a negligent Diffidence they deceive themselves and let slip the golden Opportunities of recovering by a diligent Struggle what could not be cur'd by the Use of Medicine alone.

But to give you a just and rational Idea of its Power of moving and actuating upon the Body, let us consider the whole human System as a Compound of Tubes and Glands, or to use a more rustick Phrase, a Bundle of Pipes and Strainers, fitted to one another after so wonderful a Manner as to make a proper Engine for the Soul to work with. This Description does not only comprehend the Bowels, Bones, Tendons, Veins, Nerves, and Arteries, but every Muscle and every Ligature, which is a Composition of Fibres, that are so many imperceptable Tubes or Pipes interwoven on all Sides with invisible Glands and Strainers.

This general Idea of a human Body, without considering it in the Niceties of Anatomy; let us see how absolutely necessary Labour is for the right Preservation of it. There must be frequent Motions and Agitations to mix, digest, and separate the Juices contained in it, as well as to clear and cleanse that Infinitude of Pipes and Strainers of which it is composed, and to give their solid Parts a more firm and lasting Tone; Exercise ferments the Humours, casts them into their proper Channels, throws off Redundancies, and helps Nature in those secret Distributions, without which the Body cannot subsist in Vigour, nor act with Chearfulness. I might here mention the Effects which this has upon the Soul, upon all the Faculties of the Mind, by keeping the Understanding clear, the Imagination untroubled, and refining those Spirits that are necessary for the proper Execution of our intellectual Faculties, during the present Laws of Union between Soul and Body.

It is a Neglect in this Particular, that we must ascribe the Spleen, which is so frequent in Men of studious and sedentary Tempers; as well as the Vapours, to which those of the other Sex are so often subject.

Had not Exercise been absolutely necessary for our Well-being, Nature would not have made the Body so proper for it, by giving such an Activity to the Limbs, and such a Pliancy to every Part, as necessarily produce those Compressions, Extensions, Contortions, Dilatations, and all other Kind of Motions that are necessary for the Preservation of such a System of Tubes and Glands as has been before mentioned.

And that we might not want Inducements to engage us in such an Exercise of the Body as is proper for its Welfare, it is so ordered, that nothing valuable can be procur'd without it. Not to mention Riches and Honour, even Food and Raiment are not to be come at without the Toil of the Hands, and Sweat of the Brows.

Providence furnishes us with Materials, but expects we should work them up ourselves. The Earth must be labour'd before it gives Encrease; and when it is forced into its several Products, how many Hands must they pass thro' before they are fit for Use? Manufactures, Trade, and Agriculture naturally employ more than nineteen Parts of the Species in twenty; and as for those who are not obliged to labour, by the Condition in which they are born, they are more miserable than the rest of Mankind, unless they indulge themselves in that voluntary Labour call'd Exercise, of which there is no Kind I would so recommend to both Sexes, as that of Rideing; as there is none that conduces so much to Health, and is every Way accommodated to the Body. Dr. *Sydenham* is very lavish in its Praises, and if you would learn the mechanical Effects of it described at length, you may find it learnedly treated of by Dr. *Fuller*, in a late Treatise, intituled, *Medicina Gymnastica*, or, *The Power of Exercise*. And here Mr. *Dryden*:

The first Physicians by Debauch were made;
Excess began, and Sloth sustain'd the Trade.
By Chase our long-liv'd Fathers earn'd their Food,
Toil strung the Nerves, and purified the Blood;
But we their Sons, a pamper'd Race of Men,
Are dwindled down to threescore Years and ten.
Better to hunt in Fields for Health unbought,
Than fee the Doctor for a nauseous Draught.
The Wise for Cure on Exercise depend;
God never made his Work for Man to mend.

General Maxims

FOR

HEALTH:

OR,

RULES to preserve the Body to a good old Age.

I.

IT is not good to eat too much, or fast too long, or do any thing else that is preternatural.

II.

Whoever eats or drinks too much, will be sick.

III.

If thou art dull and heavy after Meat, it's a Sign thou hast exceeded the due Measure, for Meat and Drink ought to refresh the Body, and make it chearful, not to dull and oppress it.

IV.

If thou findest those ill Symptoms, consider whether too much Meat or Drink occasions it, or both, and abate by little and little, 'till thou findest the Inconveniency remov'd.

V.

Pass not immediately from a disorder'd Life, to a strict and precise Life, but by degrees abate the Excess, for ill Customs arrive by degrees, and so must be wore off.

VI.

As to the Quality of the Food, if the Body be of a healthful Constitution, and the Meat does thee no Harm, it matters little what it is; but all Sorts must be avoided that does Prejudice, though it please the Taste never so much.

VII.

After Diet is obtain'd, the Appetite will require no more than Nature hath need of, it will desire as Nature desires.

VIII.

Old Men can fast easily; Men of ripe Age can fast almost as much, but young People and Children can hardly fast at all.

IX.

Let ancient People eat Panada, made of Bread, and Flesh Broth, which is of light Digestion; an Egg now and then will do well.

X.

Growing Persons have a great deal of Natural Heat, which requires a great deal of Nourishment, else the Body will pine.

XI.

It must be examin'd what Sort of Persons ought to feed once or twice a Day, more or less; Allowance being always made to the Person, to the Season of the Year, to the Place where one lives, and to Custom.

XII.

The more you feed foul Bodies, the more you hurt your selves.

XIII.

He that studies much, ought not to eat so much as those that work hard, his Digestion being not so good.

XIV.

The near Quantity and Quality being found out, it is safest to be kept to.

XV.

Excess in all other things whatever, as well as in Meat and drink, are to be avoided; excessive Heats and Colds, violent Exercises, late Hours, and Women, unwholsome Air, violent Winds, the Passions, *&c.*

XVI.

Youth, Age, and Sick require a different Quantity.

XVII.

And so do those of different Complexions, for that which is too much for a Phlegmatick Man, is not sufficient for the Cholerick.

XVIII.

The Measure of the Food ought to be proportionable to the Quality and Condition of the Stomach, because the Stomach is to digest it.

XIX.

The Quantity that is sufficient, the Stomach can perfectly concoct, and answers to the due Nourishment of the Body.

XX.

Hence it appears we may eat a greater Quantity of some Viands than of others of a more hard Digestion.

XXI.

The Difficulty lies in finding out an exact Measure; but eat for Necessity not Pleasure; for Lust knows not where Necessity ends.

XXII.

Wouldst thou enjoy a long Life, a healthy Body, and a vigorous Mind, and be acquainted also with the wonderful Works of God, labour in the first Place to bring thy Appetite to Reason.

XXIII.

Beware of Variety of Meats, and such as are curiously and daintily drest, which destroy a multitude of People; they prolong Appetite four times beyond what Nature requires, and different Meats are of different Natures, some are sooner digested than others, whence Crudities proceed, and the whole Digestion depraved.

XXIV.

Keep out of the Sight of Feasts and Banquets as much as may be, for it is more difficult to retain good Cheer, when in Presence, than from the Desire of it when it is away; the like you may observe in all the other Senses.

XXV.

Fancy that Gluttony is not good and pleasant, but filthy, evil, and detestable; as it really is.

XXVI.

The richest Food, when concocted, yields the most noisom Smells; and he that works and fares hard, hath a sweeter and pleasanter Body than the other.

XXVII.

Winter requires somewhat a larger Quantity than Summer; hot and dry Meats agree best with Winter, cold and moist with Summer; in Summer abate a little of your Meat and add to your Drink, and in Winter substract from your Drink and add to your Meat.

XXVIII.

If a Man casually exceeds, let him fast the next Meal and all may be well again, provided it be not often done; or if he exceed at Dinner, let him rest from, or make a slight Supper.

XXIX.

Use now and then a little Exercise a Quarter of an Hour before Meals, or swing your Arms about with a small Weight in each Hand, to leap, and the like, for that stirs the Muscles of the Breast.

XXX.

Shooting in the long Bow, for the Breast and Arms.

XXXI.

Bowling, for the Reins, Stone and Gravel, *&c.*

XXXII.

Walking, for the Stomach: And the great *Drusus* having weak and small Thighs and Legs, strengthened them by Riding, and especially after Dinner.

XXXIII.

Squinting and a dull Sight are amended by Shooting.

XXXIV.

Crookedness, by Swinging and hanging upon the Arms.

XXXV.

A temperate Diet frees from Diseases; such are seldom ill, but if they are surprized with Sickness, they bear it better, and recover it sooner, for all Distempers have their Original from Repletion.

XXXVI.

A temperate Diet arms the Body against all external Accidents, so that they are not so easily hurt by Heat, Cold, or Labour; if they at any Time should be prejudiced, they are more easily cured, either of Wounds, Dislocations, or Bruises; it also resists Epidemical Diseases.

XXXVII.

It makes Mens Bodies fitter for any Employments; it makes Men to live long; *Galen*, with many others, lived by it a Hundred Years.

XXXVIII.

Galen saith, That those that are weak-complexioned from their Mothers Womb, may (by the Help of this Art, which prescribes the coarse Diet) attain to extreme old Age, and that without Diminution of Senses or Sickness of Body; and he saith, that though he never had a healthful Constitution of Body from his Birth, yet by using a good Diet after the Twenty-seventh Year of his Age, he never fell into Sickness, unless now and then into a One Days Fever, taken by One Days Weariness.

XXXIX.

A sober Diet makes a Man die without Pain; it maintains the Senses in Vigour; it mitigates the Violence of Passions and Affections.

XL.

It preserves the Memory; it helps the Understanding; it allays the Heat of Lust; it brings a Man to that weighty Consideration of his latter End.

A

DISCOVERY

Of some

Remarkable ERRORS

In the late WRITINGS of Dr. *Mead*, *Quincey*, *Bradley*, &c. on the Plague.

The great Apprehensions that all *Europe* has received from the dreadful and raging Plague which has lately destroyed the greatest Part of the Inhabitants of *Marseilles*, has given that just Alarm to our Ministry, who under the Direction of His Majesty, by their wise and prudent Management, to the Duty of Publick Prayers, with that of a General and Solemn Fast throughout the Kingdom, have not been wanting, as much as possible, to prevent that direful Contagion which now threatens, and might be brought amongst us by the Sailors, or by Merchandize comeing from Places that are infected; and have ordered a strict Quarentine to be observed by all Ships in all the Maritime Ports liable to that Invasion.

And to be Assistant to so great a Work, the Neglect of which the Lives of the Nation being at stake, we have some the most eminent of the Physicians now in Vogue, who from that Duty to their Profession, and their Zeal to the Publick Good, have publish'd some Essays, not only of the Nature, Cause, Symptoms, Prognosticks, and Affections of this fatal Distemper; but likewise of the proper Means to be used in preventing, and fortifying against, with the proper Applications of recovering those that are seiz'd by this fatal Enemy to Mankind. Books of this kind lately published are, a short Discourse concerning Pestilential Contagion, by Dr. *Mead.* The Plague of *Marseilles* consider'd by Dr. *Bradley.* Dr. *Hodges*'s Loimologia of the Plague in *London, Anno* 1665; reprinted by Dr. *Quincy.* To which is added, an Essay of his own, with Remarks of the Infection now in *France.* To those worthy Gentlemen are we indebted for their ready Help, to their philosophical Enquiries, their learned and analytical Explanations in all the Stages of this raging Ill; and farther, by what physical Power it corrupts the Blood, destroys the Spirits, and is follow'd by Death at the last.

The Apologies that are made in their Preface, *viz.* of a short Warning, of their little Leisure, the Uncorrectness of Style, and the Typographical Errors should be favourably construed from so great an Aim of doing the Publick

———Quis talia fundo
temperet à lacrymis?———

About the Beginning of *September* the Disease was at the Height, in the Course of which Month more than Twelve thousand died in a Week[4] but from this Time its Force began to relax; and about the Close of the Year, that is, at the Beginning of *November*, People grew more healthful, and such a different Face was put upon the Publick, that although the Funerals were yet frequent, yet many who had made most haste in retiring, made the most to return, and came into the City without Fear; insomuch that in *December* they crowded back as thick as they fled; and although the Contagion had carried off, as some computed, about One hundred thousand People; after a few Months this Loss was hardly discernable.

The Doctor himself comes to no determinate Number of those that died of this Distemper, but in the Table that he has writ of the Funerals in the several Parishes within the Bills of Mortality of the Cities of *London* and *Westminster* for the Year 1665, he tells you, 68596 died of the Plague. Dr. *Mead* in the same Year 1665, that it continued in this City about ten Months, and swept away 97306 Persons. Dr. *Bradley*, in his Table from the 27th of *December*, 1664/5, takes no notice of any buried of that Distemper, but of one on the 14th of *February* following, and two on *April* the 25th, and in all, to the 7th of *June*, 89. The next following Months, to *October* the 3d, there were buried 49932, in all 50021. Why he should here break up from giving any further Account may be from the Weakness of his Intelligence, which so widely differs from all other Accounts; and in this one, with Dr. *Hodges*, who tells you, that about the Beginning of *September*, at which Time the Disease was at the Height, in the Course of which Month, more than 12000 Persons died in a Week: Whereas in *Bradley*, the most that were buried in one Week, *i. e.* from the 12th of *September* to the 19th, amounted to no more than 7165. But computing after the Manner of Dr. *Hodges*, we find (taking one Week with another, from *August* the 29th to the 27th of *September*, the Time of its greatest Fury) the exact Number of 6555; which falls short very near to one half of the Number accounted to be buried of that Distemper by Dr. *Hodges*; and we have abundant Reason to believe, that the greatest Account hitherto mentioned, may be short of the Number dying of that Distemper. If we do but observe the strict Order then published to shut up all infected Houses, to keep a Guard upon them Day and Night, to withhold from them all Manner of Correspondence from without; and that after their Recovery, to perform a Quarentine of 40 Days, in which Space if anyone else of the Family should be taken with that Distemper, the Work to be renewed again; by which tedious Confinement of the Sick and Well together, it often proved the Cause of the Loss of the Whole.

These, besides many other great Inconveniencies, were sufficient to affright the People from making the Discovery, and we may be certain, that many died of the Plague which were returned to the Magistracy under another Denomination, which might easily be obtained from the Nurses and Searchers, whether from their Ignorance, Respect, Love of Money, *&c.*

And if they vary so much in their Computation of those that died; we shall find them as widely different in the Time when 'tis said the Plague first began.

The great Dr. *Mead* on this important Subject, may establish by his Name whatever he lays down, with the same Force and Authority as the Ancients held of that *ipse dixit* of Aristotle; but as that great Master of Nature was not exempt from slipping into some Errors, *& humanum est errare*, it can be no Shock to the Reputation of this Gentleman, if we shall find him no less fallible than of some others of the Faculty who has treated on this Subject; and to this part of the time when 'tis said the Plague first began. Doctor *Mead*, by what Information he has not thought fit to tell us, does affirm, That its Beginning was in *Autumn* before the Year 1664/5; whereas Dr. *Hodges* says, in the very first Page of his *Lіomologia*, that it was not till the Close of the Year 1664; at that Season two or three Persons died suddenly in one Family at *Westminster*, of which he gives a further Light from his visiting the first Patient in the *Christmas* Holidays, and fully confirmed by the Weekly Bills of Mortality, whose first Account of those who died of the Plague were from *December* the 27th, 1664/5.

As those Gentlemen have forfeited their Infallibility by what I have proved hitherto against them, we have further Reason to suspect, whether or not the late Plague in 1665 was occasioned by that Bale of Cotton imported from *Turkey* to *Holland*, and thence to *England*, as Dr. *Hodges* makes irrefregable, and Dr. *Mead*'s Authority indisputable; which is no less a Subject of Wonder and Admiration how many Years we have escaped from the Plagues that have happened and are frequent in so many Parts of *Turkey*; as at *Grand Cairo*, which is seldome or never free from that Distemper, at *Alexandria*, *Rosetta*, *Constantinople*, *Smyrna*, *Scanderoon*, and *Aleppo*, from which Places we have the most considerable Import of any of our Neighbours, and of such Goods as are most receptive of those infectious Seeds, such as Cotton, Raw Silk, Mohair, *&c.* And though Coffee may seem less dangerous, from its Quality of being more able to resist its pestilential Effluvia, yet from the many Coverings the Bales are wrapped in, it is not hard to conceive the contagious Power might be latent in some Part of the Packidge; which Escape is the more surprising and to be wondred at from the great Encrease of our Trade and Shipping which yearly arrive from those Countries; and yet to be preserved from the like Misfortune near to this 60 Years.

Gockelius informs us, [5]"That the Contagion in the same Year 1665 was brought into *Germany* by a Body of Soldiers returning from the Wars in *Hungary* against the *Turks*, spread the Infection about *Ulm* and *Ausburgh*, where he then lived, and besides the Plague, they brought along with them the *Hungarian* and other malignant Fevers, which diffused themselves about the Neighbourhood, whereof many died.[6]

And with Submission to the wise Judgment and Opinion of these learned *Triumviri*, who have cited no fuller Authority for this Assertion than a bare Relation of it from *Hodges de Peste*; it may be no unreasonable Conjecture to have its first Progress from *Hungary*, *Germany*, and to *Holland*, from which last Place they all have agreed we certainly received the Contagion; and that we have had the Plague convey'd to us by the like Means may be found in the *Bibliotheca Anotomica*, being brought to us by some Troops from *Hungary* sent thither against the *Turks* by *Henry* VI. King of *England*.

Dr. *Mead*, who thinks it necessary to premise somewhat in general concerning the Propagation of the Plague, might, to the three Causes he has laid down, of a bad Air, diseased Persons, and Goods transported from Abroad, have added the Aliment or Diet, because affording Matter to the Juices it does not less contribute to the Generation of Diseases: And it may be observed, that in the Year before the pestilential Sickness, there was a great Mortality amongst the Cattel from a very wet Autumn, and their Carcasses being sold amongst the ordinary People at a very mean Price, a great many putred Humours might proceed from thence; and this, in the Opinion of many, was the Source of our late Calamities, when it was observed this fatal Destroyer raged with greater Triumph over the common People: And the feeding on unripened and unsound Fruits are frequently charged with a Share in Mischiefs of this Kind. *Galen*[7] is very positive in this Matter, and in one Place accuses[8] his great Master to *Hippocrates* with neglecting the Consequence of too mean a Diet: From this 'tis generally observed, that a Dearth or Famine is the Harbinger to a following Plague. And we have an Account from our Merchants trading to *Surat*, *Bencoli*, and some other Parts of the *East-Indies*, that the Natives are never free from that Distemper, which is imputed to their low and pitiful Fare. The *Europeans*, especially the *English*, escaping by their better Diet, by feeding on good Flesh, and drinking of strong generous Wine, which secures them from the Power of that Malignancy.

Their Hypotheses as widely differ in the very Substance or Nature of the Pestilence; and Dr. [9]*Hodges*, [10]*Mead*, and [11]*Quincey*, have asserted, that it proceeds from a Corruption of the Volatile Salts, or the Nitrous Spirit in the Air.

Dr. [12]*Bradley*, from the Number of poisonous Animals, Insects, or Maggots which at that Time are swimming or driving in the circumambient Air; and being sucked into our Bodies along with our Breath, are sufficiently capable of causing those direful Depredations on Mankind called the Plague. Both these Opinions are supported by the Authorities of Learned Men.

And if *Hodges*, *&c.* have the Suffrages of the greatest of the ancient Physicians, with those of *Wolfius*, *Agricola*, *Forestus*, *Fernelius*, *Belini*, *Carolus de là Font*, *&c. Bradley* may challenge to him the famed *Kirchir*, *Malhigius*, *Leeuwenhooch*, *Morgagni*, *Redi*, and *Mangetus*.

It is almost endless as well as altogether needless, to cite all the Authorities for the different Opinions, that might be collected from the most remote Antiquity down to the present Age.

And although it is yet to be contested, and might be held an occult Quality with those learned Gentlemen, we shall find, each Doctor passes his favourite Opinion upon the World with as much Infallibility as a Demonstration in *Euclid*.

[13]And for that Opinion of the famous *Kirchir*, about animated Worms, (says *Hodges*) 'I must confess I could never come at any such Discovery with the Help of the best Glasses, nor ever found the same discovered by any other; but perhaps in our cloudy Island we are not so sharp-sighted as in the serene Air of *Italy*; and with Submission to so great a Name, it seems to me very disconsonant to Reason, that such a pestilential Seminium, which is both of a nitrous and poisonous Nature, should produce a living Creature.' And he is well assured, that he is in the right, when he says, '[14]Every one of those Particulars are as clear as the Light at Noon-Day; and those Explications are so obvious to be met with in the Writings of the Learned, that it would be lost Labour to insist upon any such Thing here.'

[15]Dr. *Mead* chimes in here very tuneably with *Hodges*, and is pleased to say, 'That some Authors have imagined Infection to be performed by the Means of Insects, the Eggs of which may be conveyed from Place to Place, and make the Disease when it comes to be hatch'd. As this is a Supposition grounded upon no Manner of Observation, so I think there is no need to have Recourse to it.'

Dr. *Bradley*, who hatches this Distemper by the smaller Kind of Insects floating in the Air, is greatly jealous of his favourite Egg, from which that fatal Cockatrice breaks forth and disperses Death in every Quarter: He may be seen to promote this Hypothesis in that Discourse of his new Improvement of Planting, *&c.* and with no less Pursuit in his late Pamphlet on the Plague at *Marseilles*; where in his Preface, *p.* 13, he tells you, 'That to suppose this malignant Distemper is occasioned by Vapours only arising from the Earth, is to lay aside our Reason, *&c.*'

And it may be farther observed, That they are as remote from their Consent to one another, as in the distant Place from whence they would trace its Origin.

[16]Dr. *Mead*, from a bare Transcription of *Matthæus Villanus*, does affirm, That the Plague in the Year 1346, had its first Rise in *China*, advancing through the *East-Indies*, *Syria*, *Turkey*, *&c.* and by Shipping from the *Levant*, brought into *Europe*, which in the Year 1349. seized *England*. This is directly against Dr. *Bradley*,[17] who suggests the Plague is no where to be found in *India*, *China*, the South Parts of *Africa* and *America*, and has taken the Pains in filling up three Pages in the Defence of this Assertion.

It would be well if their Opposition ended here; but when it affects us more near, when their Difference becomes more wide in the very Means of our Preservation, and what by one is laid down as a soveraign and real Good, to be returned by another as the most fatal and destructive, is a Weight of no small Consequence, nor a less melancholly Reflection, if it should please God to inflict us with the same Calamities.

And as to those preservative Means which the Government have only a Power to direct, the making of large Fires in the Streets, as has been practised in the Times of Contagion, is a Point largely contested.

Dr. *Hodges*[18] seems inveterate against this Custom, and tells us, 'That before three Days were expired after the Fires made in 1665, the most fatal Night ensued, wherein more than 4000 expired; the Heavens both mourn'd so many Funerals, and wept for the fatal Mistake, so as to extinguish even the Fires with their Showers. May Posterity, (says he) be warned by this Mistake, and not like Empericks, apply a Remedy where they are ignorant of the Cause.'

And Dr. *Mead*[19] has an Eye to this Remark, when he tells us, 'The fatal Success of the Trials in the last Plague is more than sufficient to discourage any farther Attempts of this Nature.' Whereas on the contrary, the making of Fires in the Streets were practised from the greatest Antiquity, and supported by *Mayerne*, *Butler*, and *Harvey* in the two great Plagues before the Year 1665, and recommended by Dr. *Quincey*[20] for the Dissipation of Pestilential Vapours, *&c.* And without all manner of Dispute, Dr. *Bradley*[21] must be wholly on his Side, when he tells us, 'That the Year 1665, was the last that we can say raged in *London*, which might happen from the Destruction of the City by Fire the following Year 1666, and besides the destroying of the Eggs or Seeds of those poisonous Animals that were then in the stagnating Air, might likewise purifie the Air in such a Manner as to make it unfit for the Nourishment of others of the same kind, which were swimming or driving in the circumambient Air.'

What has been said of Fires is likewise to be understood of firing of Guns, which some have too rashly advised. Says Dr. *Mead*[22], 'The proper Correction of the Air would be to make it fresh and cool.' And here quotes from the Practice of the *Arabians* out of *Rhazes de re Medica*, &c. Dr. *Quincey*[23] 'That as the Air being still and as it were stagnate at such Times, and as it favours the Collection of poisonous Effluvia, and aggravates Infection, thinks it more effectual to let off small Parcels of the common *Pulvis Fulminans*, which must afford a greater Shock to the Air by its Explosion than by the largest Pieces of Ordnance.' In favour of which last Assertion, the Experience both of Soldiers, will justifie the firing of great Guns and Ordnance, which is frequently used in Camps, for the Dissipation of the collected pestilential Atoms, which by Concussion as well as its constituent Parts of Nitre and Sulphur, tend greatly to the Purification of the grosser Atmosphere within the Compass of their Activity; and by the Seamen in their Voyages in the Southern Parts of the World, when sometimes the Air is so gross, and hangs so low upon them, as to be almost suffocated. And in the late Plague at *Marseilles* the constant firing of great Guns at Morning and Evening, by the Appointment of *Monsieur le Marquis de Langeron* their Governour, was esteemed of great Relief to the Inhabitants.

Nay, their Contest will not end in a Pipe of Tobacco, against which Dr. *Hodges*[24] declares himself a profess'd Enemy: 'But whether (says he) we regard the narcotick Quality of this *American* Henbane; or the poisonous Oil which exhales from it in Smoaking, or that prodigious Discharge of Spittle which it occasions, and which Nature wants for many other important Occasions, besides the Aptitude of the pestilential Poison to be taken down along with it; he chose rather to supply its Place with Sack.'

Dr. *Bradley*[25] redeems it from this low Character, and represents it as a great Antidote in the last Plague *Anno* 1665. 'The Distemper did not reach those who smoak'd Tobacco every Day, but particularly it was judged best to smoak in a Morning: He farther gives you an Account of a famous Physician, who in the pestilential Time took every Morning a Cordial to guard his Stomach, and after that a Pipe or two, before he went to visit his Patients; at the same time he had an Issue in his Arm, by which, when it begun to smart, he knew he had received some Infection (as he says) and then had recourse to his Cordial and his Pipe.' By this Means only he preserved himself, as several others did at that Time by the same Method.

I could heartily wish those worthy Gentlemen had struck in with greater Harmony to the Satisfaction and Security of the People, whose Expectations were greatly raised by the Hopes of their Assistance, by gaining a greater

Light into the Nature, Quality, Symptoms, and Affections of this definitive Ill, to have promoted their Safety, by giving the necessary Indications relating to the Cure, as well as the necessary Precautions in order to guard us from that secret Attack which may approach us by very minute and unheeded Causes; the which, from their different Notions and positive Contradictions, lay too deep from the narrow Re-searches of those Philosophizing and Learned Gentlemen, and for the Manner whereby it kills, its Approaches are generally so secret, that Persons seiz'd with it seem to be fallen into an Ambuscade or a Snare, of which there was no Manner of Suspicion. And there are very few Discourses relating to the Pestilence but what abound in many Instances of this kind: And the Learned *Boccace*, in his Admirable Description of the Plague at *Florence* (quoted by Dr. *Mead*[26] *Anno* 1348) relates what himself saw, 'That two Hogs finding in the Streets some Rags which had been thrown off from a poor Man dead of the Disease, after snuffling upon them, and tearing them with their Teeth, fell into Convulsions, and died in less than an Hour.'

The Misfortune which happened in the Island of *Bermudas* about 25 Years since, which Account is from Dr. *Halley*; A Sack of Cotton put ashore by Stealth, lay above a Month without any Prejudice to the People of the House where it was hid; but when it came to be distributed among the Inhabitants, it carried such a Contagion along with it, that the Living scarce sufficed to bury the Dead.

And Dr. *Quincey*[27] has somewhere read a strange Story in *Baker*'s Chronicle, 'of a great Rot amongst Sheep, which was not quite rooted out until about Fourteen Years time, that was brought into *England* by a Sheep bought for its uncommon Largeness, in a Country then infected with the same Distemper.'

Fracastorius[28], an eminent *Italian* Physician, tells us, 'That in the Year 1511, when the *Germans* were in Possession of *Verona*, there arose a deadly Disease amongst the Soldiers, from the wearing only of a Coat purchased for a small Value; for it was observed, that every Owner of it soon sickned and died; until at last the Cause of it was so manifestly known from some Infection in the Coat, that it was ordered to be burned.' Ten thousand Persons, he says, were computed to fall by this Plague before it ceased.

And *Kephale*, in his *Medela Pestilentiæ*, printed *Anno* 1665, acquaints us, That the following Plagues were produced from the following Causes.

That in the Year 1603, the contagious Seeds were brought to *England* amongst Seamens Clothes in *White-Chappel*; and in that Year there died of the Plague 30561.

That in the Year 1625, was bred and produced by rotten Mutton at *Stepney*; of which died 35403 Persons.

That in the Year 1630, was brought to us by a Bale of Carpets from *Turkey*, of which died 1317 Persons.

That in the Year 1636, was brought over to us by a Dog from *Amsterdam*; of which died 10400 Persons.

That in the Year 1665, was brought from *Turkey* in a Bale of Cotton to *Holland*, thence to *England*; in this great Plague died no less than 100,000 People.

And at *Marseilles*, in this present Year 1720, the Plague has swept away more than 70000 Persons, which was brought in Goods from *Sidon*, a fam'd and ancient City and Sea-port in *Phœnicia*, and the same which sometimes is mentioned in Holy Writ.

From the Neighbourhood of this last Contagion, the frightful Apprehensions of the People are rais'd to the greatest Height; and when every one is consulting his own Security, how to guard and preserve himself from that dreadful Enemy, nothing can come more seasonably to their Relief, than to lay before them a *Compendium* of the best and approved Rules for their Conduct; to which End I have carefully collected, from the successful Practice of Dr. *Glisson*, Sir *Thomas Millington*, Dr. *Charlton*, and other Learned Physicians in the last Plague, with what only may be of Use from the abounding Prescripts of those who have lately published, and as this Evil is supported throughout the general Practice, it appears to be the Result of the Reasoning of some of the Learned Sons of *Æsculapius*, to marshal into the Field as many Compositions as if only by their Number they might be able to pull down the Tyranny of this fatal Destroyer.

It would be a Work insuperable, and altogether foreign to the Method I have gone by, to extract all the Medicines which some Writers abound with for this End; it is our Business here chiefly to take Notice of that saving *Regimen*, that Rule of Self-governing, which proved more successful in the Preservation of the People in the late Plague, than all the abounding *Nostrums* that have been crouded into the Practice, the which has become a due Reproach to the Faculty.

Turpe est Doctori, quem culpa
redarguit ipsum.

And it is here worthy of our first Remark, That the last Plague, in the Year 1665, as well from the late Accounts we have of that at *Marseilles*, the poorer Sort of People were those that mostly suffered, which can only be attributed to their mean and low Fare, whereas the most nutritive and generous Diet should be promoted, and such as generate a warm and rich Blood, Plenty of Spirits, and what easily perspires, which otherwise would be apt to ferment and generate Corruption.

Your greatest Care is, to have your Meat sweet and good, neither too moist nor flashy, having a certain Regard to such as may create an easy Digestion, and observing that roasted Meats on those Occasions should be preferred; as Beef, Mutton, Lamb, Venison, Turkey, Capon, Pullet, Chicken, Pheasant, and Partridge: But Pidgeon, and most Sort of Wild and Sea Fowl to be rejected: Salt Meats to be cautiously used; all hot, dry, and spicey Seasonings to be avoided; most Pickles and rich Sauces to be encouraged, with the often Use of Garlick, Onion, and Shallot; the cool, acid, and acrid Herbs and Roots, as Lettuce, Spinnage, Cresses, Sorrel, Endive, and Sellery; all windy Things, which are subject to Putrefaction, to be refrained, as all kind of Pulse, Cabbage, Colliflower, Sprouts, Melons, Cucumbers, *&c.* as also most Summer Fruits, excepting Mulberries, Quinces, Pomegranates, Raspers, Cherries, Currants, and Strawberries, which are of Service when moderately eat of.

All light and viscid Substances to be avoided, as Pork, most Sorts of Fish, of the latter that may be eat, are Soles, Plaise, Flounder, Trout, Gudgeon, Lobster, Cray-fish, and Shrimps, no Sort of Pond-Fish being good; and for your Sauce, fresh melted Butter, or Oil mixed with Vinegar or Verjuice, the Juice of Sorrel, Pomegranates, Barberries, of Lemon or *Seville* Orange, which two last are to be preferred, from their Power of resisting all Manner of Putrefaction, as well to cool the violent Heat of the Stomach, Liver, *&c.*

For your Bread, to be light, and rather stale than new, not to drink much of Malt Liquors, avoiding that which is greatly Hopped, or too much on the ferment, Mead and Metheglin are of excellent Use, and good Wines taken moderately are a strong Preservative, Sack especially being accounted the most Soveraign and the greatest Alexipharmick: Excess is dangerous to the most healthy Constitution, which may beget Inflammations of fatal Consequence in pestilential Cases.

Let none go Home fasting, every one, as they can procure, to take something as may resist Putrefaction; some may take Garlick with Bread and Butter, a Clove two or three, or with Rue, Sage, Sorrel, dipt in Vinegar, the Spirit of Oil of Turpentine frequently drank in small Doses is of great Use; as also to lay in steep over-Night, of Sage well bruis'd two Handfuls, of Wormwood one Handful, of Rue half a Handful, put to them in an Earthen Vessel four Quarts of Mild Beer; which in the Morning to be drank fasting.

The Custom that prevails now of drinking Coffee, Bohea-Tea, or Chocolate, with Bread and Butter, is very good; at their going abroad 'tis proper to carry Rue, Angelica, Masterwort, Myrtle, *Scordianum* or Water-Germander,

Wormwood, Valerian or Setwal-Root, *Virginian* Snake-Root, or Zedoary in their Hands to smell to, or of Rue one Handful stampt in a Mortar, put thereto Vinegar enough to moisten it, mix them well, then strain out the Juice, wet a Piece of Sponge or a Toast of brown Bread therein, tie it in a Bit of thin Cloth to smell to.

But there is nothing more grateful and efficacious than the volatile *Sal Armoniac*, well impregnated with the essential Oils of aromatick Ingredients, which may be procured dry, and kept in small Bottles, from a careful Distillation of the common *Sal Volatile Oleosum.*

Sometimes more fœtid Substances agree better with some Persons than the more grateful Scents, of which the most useful Compositions may be made of Rue, Featherfew, *Galbanum*, *Assafœtida*, and the like, with the Oil of Wormwood, the Spirit or Oil drawn and dropt upon Cotton, so kept in a close Ivory Box, though with Caution to be used, the often smelling to, dilating the Pores of the Olfactory Organs, which may give greater Liberty for the pestilential Air to go along with it. A Piece of Orris Root kept in the Mouth in passing along the Streets, or of Garlick, Orange or Lemon Peel, or Clove, are of very great Service. As also Lozenges of the following Composition, which are always profitable to be used fasting; of Citron Peel two Drams, Zedoary, Angelica, of each, prepar'd in Rose Vinegar, half a Dram, Citron Seeds, Wood of Aloes, Orris, of each two Scruples, Saffron, Cloves, Nutmeg, one Scruple, Myrrh, Ambergrease, of each six Grains, Sugarcandy one Ounce; make into Lozenges with Gum Traganth and Rose-water.

I know not indeed a greater Neglect than not keeping the Body clean, and the keeping at a distance any thing superfluous and offensive, to keep the House airy and fresh, and moderately cool, and to strew it with Herbs, Rushes, and Boughs, which yield refreshing Scents, and contribute much to the purifying of the Air, and resisting the Infection; of this kind all Sorts of Rushes and Water Flags, Mint, Balm, Camomil Grass, Hyssop, Thyme, Pennyroyal, Rue, Wormwood, Southernwood, Tansy, Costmary, Lime-tree, Oak, Beech, Walnut, Poplar, Ash, Willow, *&c.* A frequent Change of Clothes, and a careful drying or airing them abroad, with whisking and cleaning of them from all Manner of Filth and Dust, which may harbour Infection, as it is likewise to keep the Windows open at Sun-Rise till the Setting, especially to the North and East, for the cold Blasts from those Quarters temper the Malignity of pestilential Airs.

Preservative Fumigations are largely talked of by all on those Occasions, and they with good Reason deserve to be practised. And of the great Number of Aromatick Roots and Woods, I should chiefly prefer Storax, Benjamin, Frankinsense, Myrrh, and Amber, the Wood of Juniper, Cypress and Cedar,

CPSIA information can be obtained
at www.ICGtesting.com
Printed in the USA
LVHW041019020323
740706LV00008B/1074

9 789356 895201